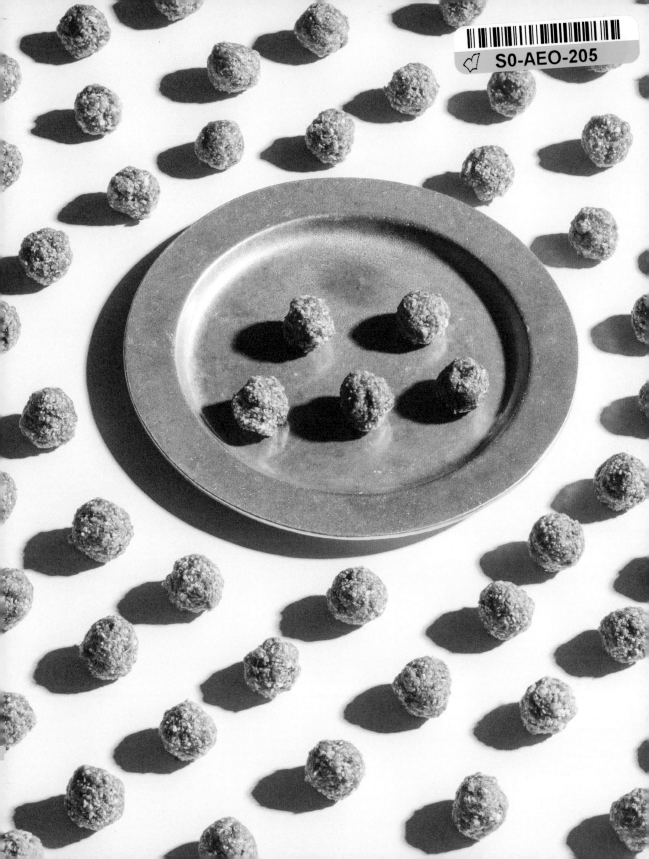

AMANDA CHANTAL BACON

THE

MOON JUICE

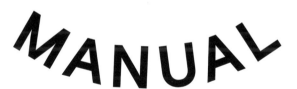

ADAPTOGENIC RECIPES FOR NATURAL STRESS RELIEF

AVERY
an imprint of Penguin Random House
New York

A
AVERY

an imprint of
Penguin Random House LLC
penguinrandomhouse.com

Most Avery books are available
at special quantity discounts
for bulk purchase for sales
promotions, premiums, fund-
raising, and educational needs.
Special books or book excerpts
also can be created
to fit specific needs.

For details, write: SpecialMarkets
@penguinrandomhouse.com

ISBN 9780593083963
eBook ISBN 9780804188234

Printed in China

10 9 8 7 6 5 4 3 2 1

Art direction and design
by Heather Scott (More Milk)

Photography by
Nastassia Brückin

The recipes contained in this
book are to be followed exactly
as written. The publisher is not
responsible for your specific
health or allergy needs that may
require medical supervision. The
publisher is not responsible for
any adverse reactions to the
recipes contained in this book.

To my husband—I got as far as I could alone;
thank you for activating this health and happiness

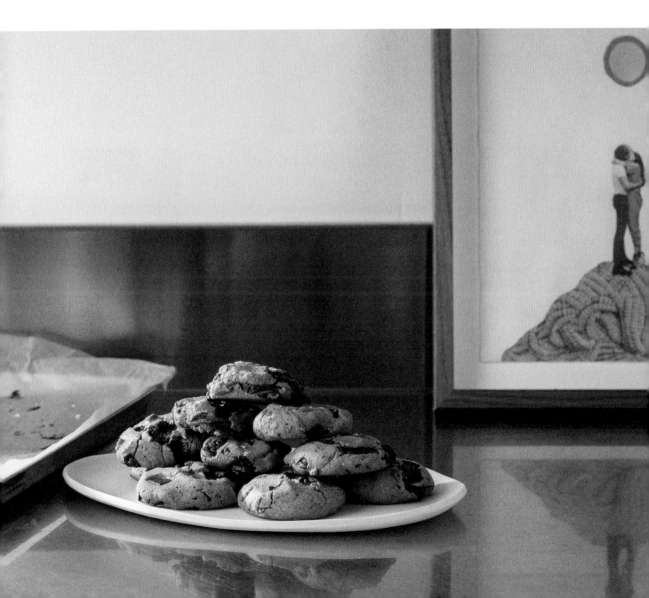

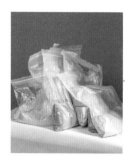
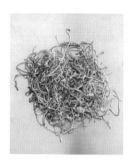
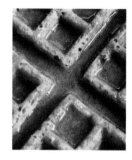
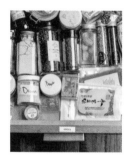
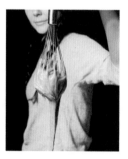

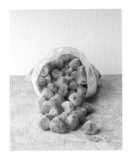

Beauty

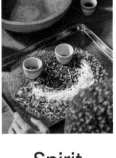

Spirit

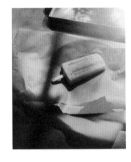

Power

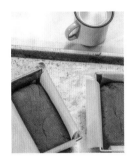

Brain

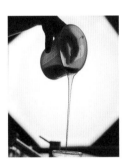

Dream

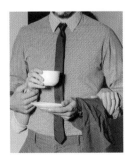

Sex

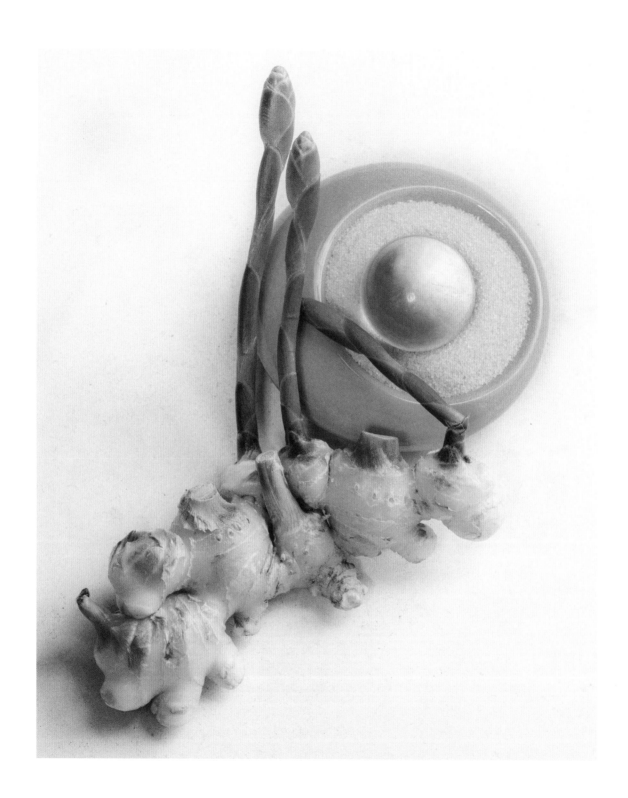

Advisory Board

I called upon the best functional medicine doctors and nutritionists to get their perspective.

Dr. Pratima Raichur combines the wisdom of Ayurveda with her expertise as a chemist, botanist, aesthetician, and ayurvedic doctor, and is the author of *Absolute Beauty*.

Dr. Mark Hyman is a family physician, the director of the Cleveland Clinic Center for Functional Medicine, founder and medical director of the UltraWellness Center, chairman of the board of the Institute for Functional Medicine, and a ten-time *New York Times* bestselling author.

Dr. Frank Lipman is board certified in internal medicine, and integrates acupuncture, Chinese medicine, functional medicine, nutrition, and herbal medicine into his practice. He is a *New York Times* bestselling author of five books.

Dr. Sarah Gottfried is a Harvard-educated physician-scientist and an MIT-trained bioengineer and is board certified in obstetrics and gynecology. She is a systems-based hormone expert and the *New York Times* bestselling author of *Younger*, *The Hormone Reset Diet*, and *The Hormone Cure*.

Alisa Vitti, HHC, is a functional nutritionist, AADP, best-selling author of *WomanCode*, and the founder of FLOLiving.com, a virtual health center that supports women's hormonal and reproductive health.

Maya Shetreat-Klein, MD, is an integrative pediatric neurologist based in New York City, herbalist, and author of *The Dirt Cure*.

THE

ADAPTOGEN

KINGDOM

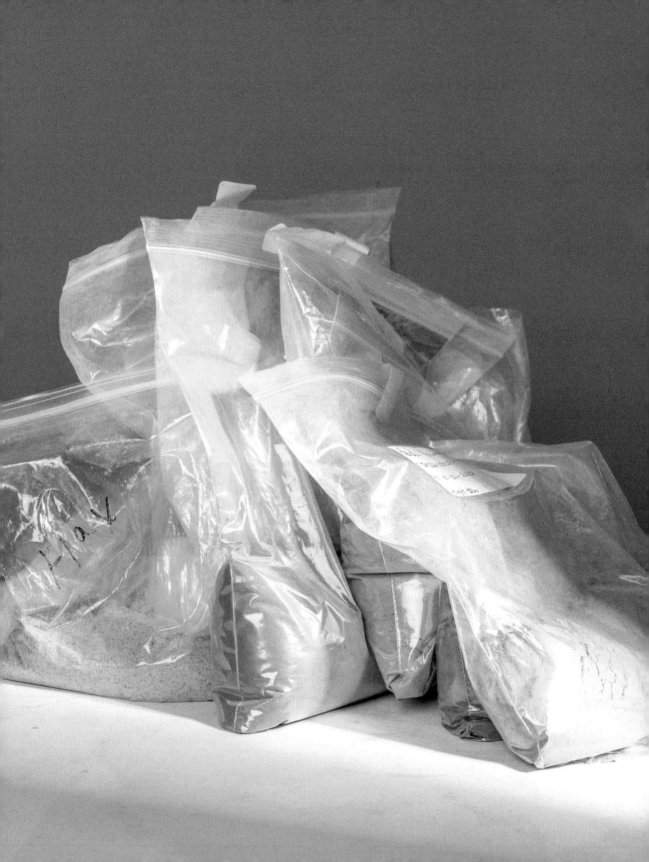

Welcome to
the Adaptogen Kingdom

I'm Amanda, the founder of Moon Juice, a resource for healing. This book is not about floating through days in a field of wildflowers sipping a golden latte; that is not what my life looks like. I, like you, am a real person. I'm a mother, wife, and CEO of a growing company that I've continued to build from the ground up. I was diagnosed with an autoimmune condition over a decade ago. I have since put it into remission and now rely on easy and natural ways to manage stress on a daily basis. Before getting to the root of my issues and taking care of myself effectively, I struggled with many aspects of my physical and emotional body. I have had points in my life where I was meant to be my most fertile but didn't menstruate due to hypothyroidism. I have experienced anxiety levels that were debilitating and such energy lows that I couldn't get out of bed in the morning or function past 3 p.m. The information and ministrations in this book aren't flights of fancy for me; they've been crucial to my vitality and have encouraged a beautiful life I wasn't sure I could have. I wouldn't have found my stamina without the support of these plants called adaptogens. My life changed drastically when I started to incorporate their intelligence into my daily habits, and the ease, simplicity, and joy of adding this next layer of health to my life is something I want to share with you for these increasingly demanding times.

There was a morning, years ago, when I woke up and decided to put my energy behind feeling the absolute best that I could, and I haven't looked back. I realized that if I was going to take back my power, if I was ever going to feel like I was in the right body, if I was going to do any of the things I knew I had the capacity to do, and if I was going to find the joy I knew my heart was born to live, I

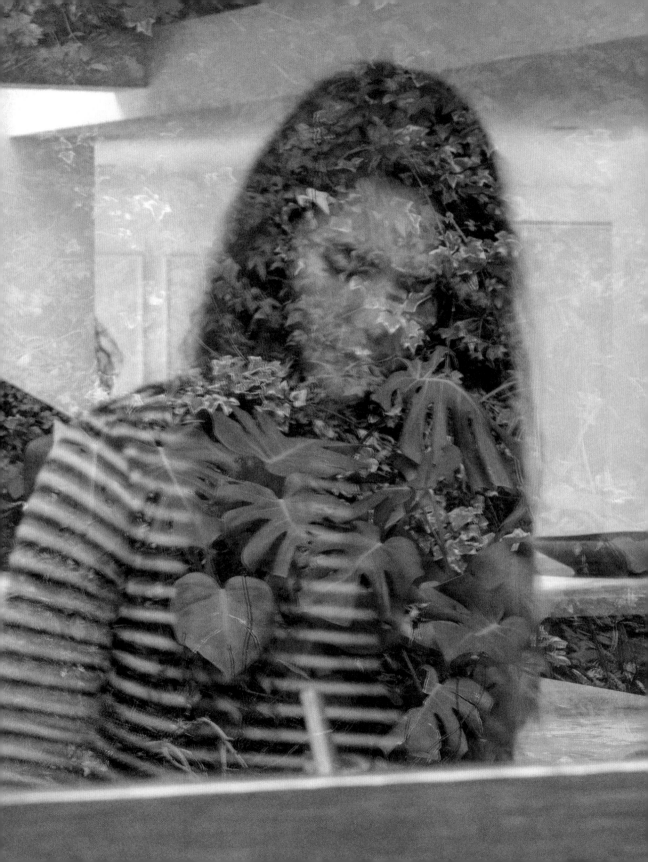

had to fundamentally change the way I took care of myself. The first step in this transformation was acknowledging that feeling sick and tired was not my truth. What I learned—through much seeking, studying, trial, and error—was that I needed to shift my diet to include foods that naturally nourish and support the body's intricate physiology; foods that tame inflammation, stabilize blood sugar, neutralize acidity, mineralize, balance hormones, regulate the biome, feed the brain, stoke the fire, and lift the spirit. This plant-forward food as medicine was ground zero for my healing, along with meditation, gentle movement, connecting more deeply to myself and others, and quality rest. But there was yet another discovery that helped me unlock new levels— phenomenal levels—of vitality and connectedness. It helped me restore my being into a fortresslike respite of calm, strength, and resilience. And it became the basis of the alchemical wellness that Moon Juice provides. This breakthrough was my journey with adaptogens.

Adaptogens are what fill all those amber glass jars on the shelves of our shops, and they're what make up the Dusts that we've become known for. When people come in looking to remedy an ailment—from sleeplessness to hormonal imbalance, brain fog to spiritual disconnect— these potent, safe, natural correctives are what we prescribe. Simply put, adaptogens are plants. They are super herbs and super mushrooms that help your body both heal from and ward off the damaging effects of stress. As we'll talk about much more throughout this book, stress is one of the most devastating aggressors to the body. It can overpower the immune system; shut down the metabolism; trigger pain; cloud the mind; kill libido; hamper fertility; and cause despair, exhaustion, and feeling overwhelmed. Oftentimes, stress stands in the way of our best efforts to take care of ourselves, whether through moving the body, preparing a healthy meal, or taking probiotics. Its effects can be dramatic and chronic, or devious and subtle. Either way, it derails our well-being.

When I talk about stress, I'm not just referring to things like deadlines or bills or inboxes jammed with demands—or even more intense forms that stress takes, such as grief, overwhelming change, and pain (emotional or physical). I'm also including stressors that we have little or no control over, like pollutants in the air and water, the amount of noise we experience, and even the artificial light in our environment. Adaptogens, as they've been used for thousands of years in healing traditions, defend you from this seemingly inevitable erosion. They aren't stimulants, but they'll give you energy. They have the power to give you stamina, calm the mind, and flood the brain with happy-making amino acids like L-dopa. They are nature's antibiotics, analgesics, and mood stabilizers. They are the great protectors of the body's physiological systems and are what give you the velocity, strength, and foresight to partake in necessary acts of self-care and world action. And yes, they also help preserve collagen protein, protect cells from free-radical damage, and balance the skin. But best of all, adaptogens give you the ability to tend to your body in an ever-evolving way. Every day, you can wake up and ask yourself, *How do I feel this morning?*—or even better, *How do I want to feel this morning?*—and know that your tailor-made treatment is just a couple of spoonfuls away in your next cup of drinking chocolate, infused honey, or batch of pancakes.

In my first book, *The Moon Juice Cookbook*, my aim was to help you become the Alchemist. I wanted to first bridge the world of healing with the pleasures and rituals of feeding yourself, then give you the tools to transform your health from the inside out. I wanted to put your hands on the reins of your own quest and connect you with your power to nourish your body into its fullest potential. There are few things I'm more passionate about than introducing people to the medicinal wonders of food and reminding them of their body's innate power to heal itself. I live in awe of the amazing knowledge that plants have and how they can transform our bodies, minds, and spirits. I eventually came to realize what exactly this book needed to be.

If *The Moon Juice Cookbook* was an adventure story about the lush wilderness of a plant-rich diet, then this book is your adaptogen field guide. It is your handbook for understanding a class of healing plants—what I like to call the Adaptogen Kingdom. The knowledge in this book comes from ancient tradition that is cofounded by science—I'm just here to organize the information, help you tune in to that space, and hack your daily habits to include these easy, effective, and delicious practices. The most important part of this is that *you* are becoming the Alchemist and the self-healer. You are the one scanning your body and mind to see what needs balancing and restoring. That clarity is what comes from understanding that you have just as much access to this herbal intelligence as anyone—and that it all starts with these plants. They will awaken, empower, and enable you to step into the natural wisdom you were born with, a connection to earth and spirit that is already alive and well inside you. Now it's just a matter of stepping over the threshold.

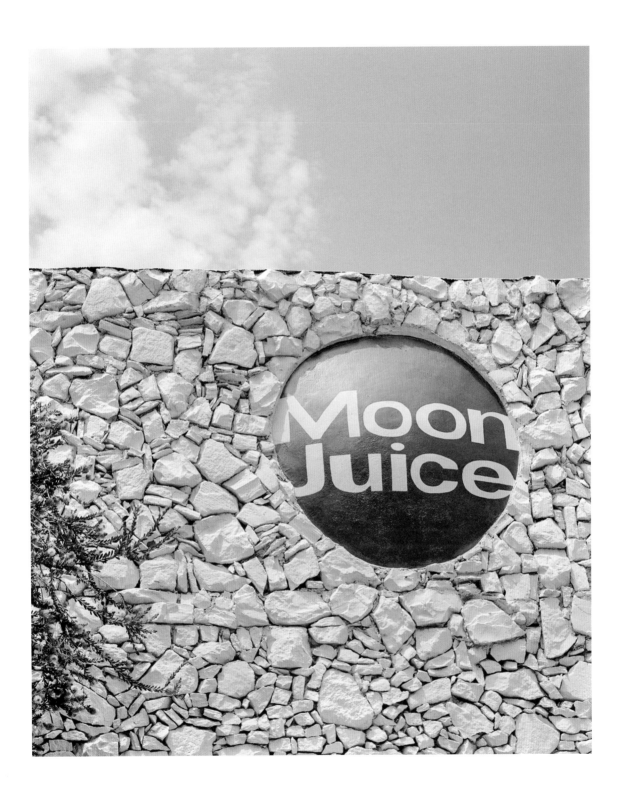

BIOLOGY FOR THE FUTURE

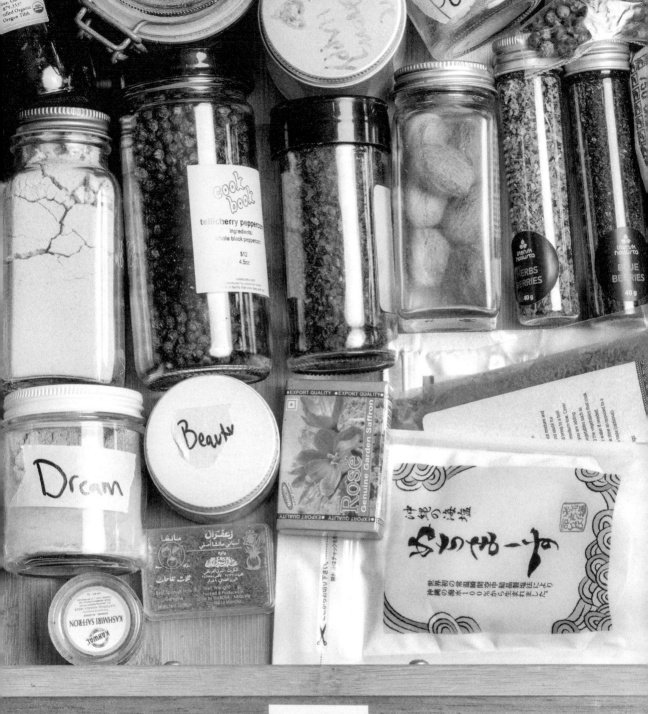

SPICES

Protecting
Your Health

When I think about wellness, I'm not just thinking about the absence of disease. I'm imagining a state of complete physical, mental, and spiritual well-being. That includes but is not limited to:

1　Tamed inflammation
2　Clarity of mind
3　Balanced hormones
4　Vibrant skin
5　Dynamic sexuality
6　Optimal immune function
7　Restful sleep
8　Reliable digestion
9　Connected spirit

That said, "healthy" is not a fixed state. It's not a goal that, once attained, never goes away, or a thing that we can acquire and put on the shelf like a trophy. It's not a distinction you automatically get from an intense thirty-day detox, and it's definitely not what's achieved by doing everything "right" or eliminating everything "bad." No matter how many plants you eat, how cultured your microbiome, how deeply and often you meditate, or how committed you are to the cause, health is still something that fluctuates with our lives, each and every day.

I'm not trying to discourage you from trying to reach your version of true, radical health (because you absolutely can and should). I'm hoping that, like me, you'll be humbled by this challenge and that you'll embrace the adventure. Because once you leave behind the notion that you have some kind of fixed destination to get to—and that there's only one way to get there—you can let go of the "should"s

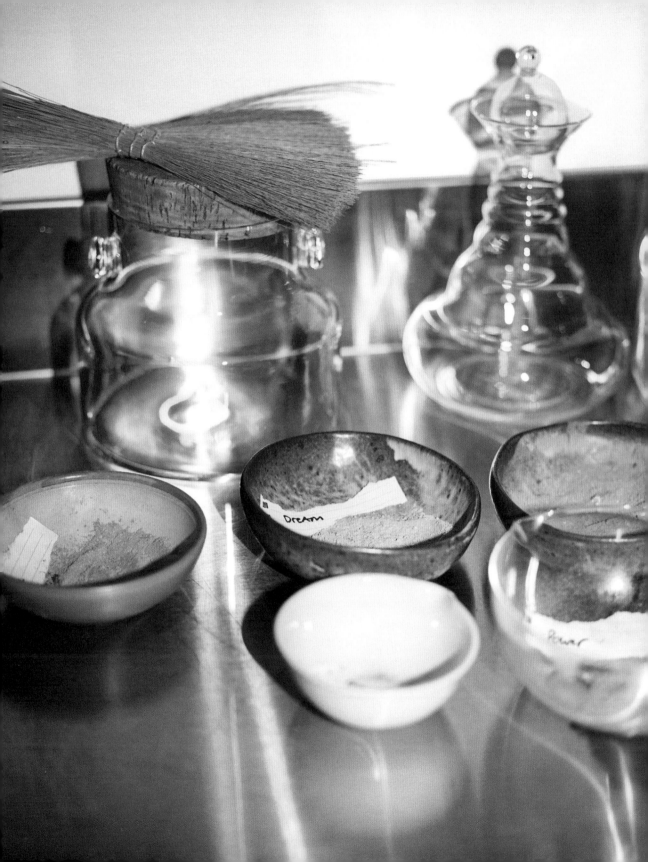

and instead wake up each morning asking yourself, *What do you need today? What can I give you to support what you need to do?* And best of all, you can stop thinking of health as this big, abstract, overwhelming thing and start having a more nuanced understanding of the physiological systems that directly influence the well-being of your body, mind, and spirit.

One of the biggest reasons we need to constantly recalibrate our internal health compass is that no matter how much control we think we have over our insides, there's a whole lot that we have no control over on the outside. There are so many aspects of our environment that tax our systems on a daily basis—driving a car, navigating crowded spaces, reading the news, or experiencing any number of emotions. And then there's the above-and-beyond like riding an airplane and constant screen time. Welcome to the now, where our bodies are experiencing things that our grandparents couldn't have even fathomed. Technology, travel, and work have evolved into a 24/7 demand. Your grandma didn't have people constantly vying for her attention through calls and texts; she wasn't on social media; maybe she wasn't juggling home and a career. Her food didn't come from engineered crops; her water and air weren't polluted with chemical toxins; and her ozone layer wasn't depleted. We also don't have the community and support that were once the norm, things that we need. There was a time when your mother, sister, grandmother, aunt, or cousins could help with raising the children. If you were pregnant or postpartum, they would be there to offer support and guidance. If you were suffering, you'd have that community for comfort and reassurance. Now, instead of coming home from a day of challenging physical labor to enjoy some restful family connection, you rush home from the office, pick up your kid, *maybe* you cook, but more likely you pull something out of the fridge, and you eat standing up while accommodating others.

Basically, compared to people who lived on this planet one hundred years ago, we're space travelers. We all have this notion that when the future gets here we'll know it because cars will fly, robots will clean, and we'll all be booking tickets to the moon. We're already there. Modern life has taken us to futuristic wilds, and yet we're expecting our physical, emotional, and spiritual selves to not be any different for it.

This is stress, an opposing force that can't be eliminated from our lives, no matter how hard we try.

Stress isn't just a mental state. It is a physical response that travels throughout your entire body. In some instances, temporary bouts of stress can be beneficial, like when you need an extra shot of energy or need to focus on a task. But when the stress response is activated too frequently or over a prolonged period of time, it can damage your organs, cells, and brain.

Stress
101

WHAT IS STRESS?

In the most basic terms, a stressor is any agent or event that threatens the body's healthy resting state, or homeostasis. Things that can stress us out include:

1   Bacteria, viruses, molds, and parasites

2   Fumes, pesticides, synthetic drugs, and heavy metals

3   Extreme cold, heat, noise, ultraviolet sunlight, altitude, allergens, and radiation

4   Food allergies, processed foods, and alcohol

5   Strenuous physical activity, surgery, trauma, too little food or sleep, and chronic overstimulation

6   Fear, anxiety, anger, and overwhelming responsibility

HOW DOES THE BODY RESPOND TO STRESS?

To understand how pervasive stress-related damage can be in the body, we have to first understand the stress reaction itself, a meticulously choreographed cascade of reactions triggered by a **perceived** (this is a key concept we will get into) threat:

The stress response starts in the **brain**, where the **amygdala** sounds the alarm and the **hypothalamus** sends word to the rest of the body.

STOP THE STRESS LOOP

1

The **adrenal glands** pump the hormone **epinephrine** (a.k.a. adrenaline) into the bloodstream. The **sympathetic nervous system**—part of your central nervous system—goes into full beast mode: your breathing intensifies as your lungs expand; your heart beats faster and raises your blood pressure; blood is redirected from the digestive tract to your heart, muscles, vital organs, and limbs; your blood sugar spikes as the body floods itself with more available energy stores; your senses sharpen; your ability to perceive pain diminishes; and you prepare to fight whatever threat there might be—or flee from it.

2

The **hypothalamus**, **pituitary gland**, and **adrenal glands** form what's called the **HPA axis**. This conglomerate wants to keep the stress response going in order to eradicate the perceived danger, so it throws fuel on the fire by stimulating the production of **cortisol**, a steroid hormone that encourages the body to stay in this amped-up state.

3

The **autonomic nervous system** joins the party. This network of nerve connections links your brain to your enteric or intestinal nervous system. (Yep, a good part of your nervous system is in your gut—more on that in a bit.) In addition to causing that funny sensation you get when you're particularly amped up or anxious, this brain-gut connection temporarily suspends digestion so you can take care of more important matters, and so that blood can service the heart and lungs.

4

When the HPA axis decides that the threat has passed, cortisol production wanes, allowing the **parasympathetic nervous system** to take over, quell the stress response, and recover.

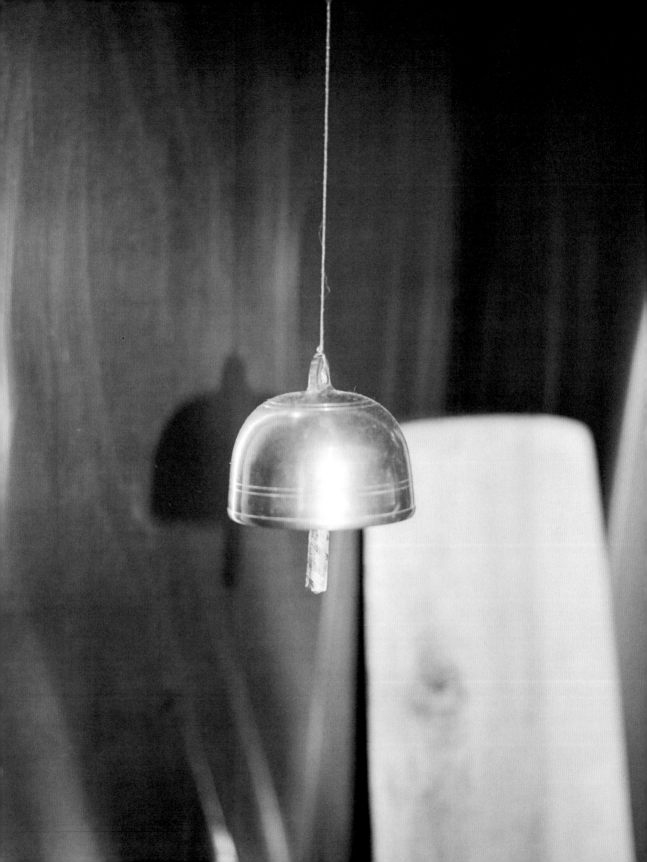

DR. PRATIMA RAICHUR

What is stress?

Stress is simply a perception of an event or feeling that begins in the mind. That said, there is no absolute or objective truth about what stress is; something that is stressful to one person may not be stressful to another, and vice versa. Once the mind labels something as "stress," the entire body responds: Adrenaline is released, senses go on alert, breathing and digestion are interrupted, blood sugar spikes to provide more energy, and the heart works harder to supply blood to the limbs. In the case of prolonged or chronic patterns of stress, the body remains in these high-alert modes. Over time, this degrades the functions of our parasympathetic nervous system, causing dysfunction in various other systems, including endocrine, digestive, respiratory, cardiovascular, immune, brain functioning, endurance/energy levels, as well as the ability of our cells to repair and rejuvenate.

DR. MARK HYMAN

What does it look like when your immune system/brain/sex drive, etc., are at peak performance?

So many of us don't know how bad we feel until we start feeling good—myself included. You have a sense of mental clarity and tasks become easier and joyful. Your immune system becomes stronger, and you might realize that you haven't been sick in a long time. When you're at peak performance, your digestion runs smoothly, you have a healthy sex drive, and you have a healthy response to stress.

What are the signs of a body in distress when it comes to how the body looks and/or feels?

The short answer is: If you don't feel that great, the body is most likely experiencing some type of distress. Craving sugar or refined carbohydrates, feeling tired and sluggish, and having joint pain or muscle aches, skin challenges such as acne or eczema, low sex drive, trouble remembering things, bloating, gas, diarrhea, or simply feeling like crap are just a few of the signs that the body is in distress. We are meant to feel good, and we definitely should not settle for anything less.

Why not just take a pill for individual maladies?

Our recurrent conventional medical model is the pursuit of a holy grail—a pill for every ill. This approach has failed and will continue to fail. The body is a system, and to treat illness, we have to treat the entire system and not just our symptoms. Using a pill for an ill is often used to just cover up the symptoms instead of getting to the root cause of disease and illness.

Why Is
Stress So Disruptive?

The body craves its particular balance. It wants a consistent temperature around 98.6 degrees, quality breath, stable levels of glucose, and alkalinity of the blood. As you move through the world, your body keeps up with external demands, working diligently to maintain that balance. It breaks down your food and allocates the nutrients and energy to maintain your personalized ecosystem by sending essential nerve impulses, pumping lymph fluid, delivering oxygen to cells, and dismantling toxins and flushing them out.

But with stress, the body goes from performing system-wide maintenance and upkeep to emergency mode. Where you once had round-the-clock care for healing injuries, patrolling for pathogens, or producing necessary hormones like restful sleep-promoting melatonin, now your body is putting out a fire that may not even be there. It's down to essentials only—your heart will keep pumping, your blood will keep flowing, and your brain will still send messages to the muscles. But with homeostasis disrupted, your body becomes vulnerable. Suddenly you may find yourself experiencing more aches and pains, fatigue, colds, allergies, and feeling a persistent sense of "blah." This kind of breakdown can happen when we don't give our body the kind of nourishing food and niceties it deserves—like getting enough rest, movement, or calm—but it can also happen to the most vigilant proponents of self-care, and I speak from experience.

The stress response has gotten us through evolution as a species. It's what gives us the superhuman reflexes to escape or confront truly dangerous situations, without even having to pause to think about it. However, these primary fear detectors and decision makers in the brain—the

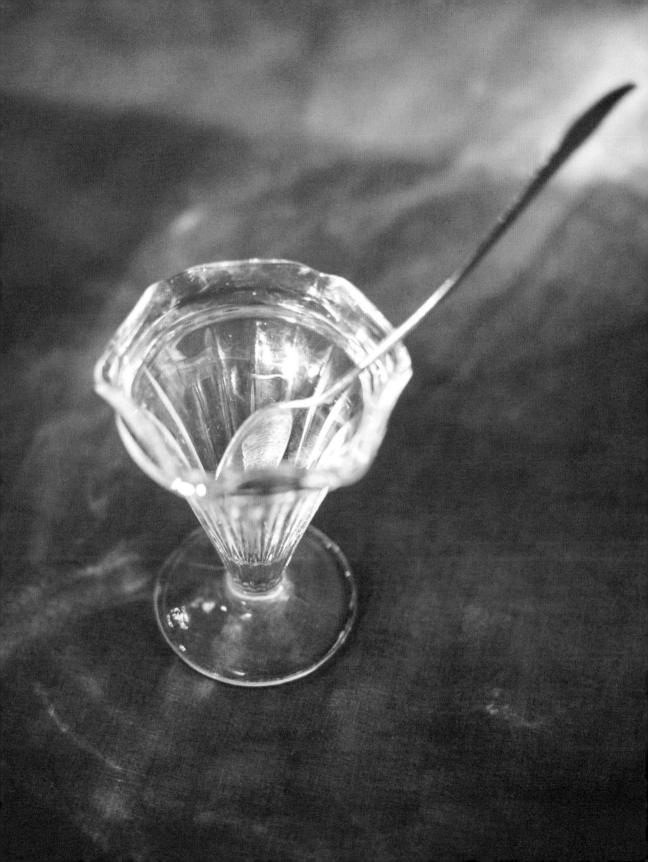

amygdala and hypothalamus—are part of a primitive construct. Many of us no longer live in a wild environment where threats loom in the foliage. Our stress response isn't tempered to account for whether or not something is truly life-threatening—an e-mail can now elicit the same body-wide red alarm as an alligator.

The other part of the equation is that while the body does have tools for soothing itself after the stress response—called the "adaptive response," or the process of reestablishing homeostasis—these are limited resources. The more stress you experience, the less adaptive energy you have. If you're constantly experiencing stress and deteriorating your adaptive energy, then your body can't recalibrate. And if your body can't recalibrate, then it can't function optimally. In order to try to keep up with demand, your body will start using more energy, desperately trying to convert nutrients to usable fuel. Plus, it will crank out increasing levels of cortisol and decreasing levels of DHEA (dehydroepiandrosterone), an adrenal hormone, which is essentially a cocktail for systemic exhaustion.

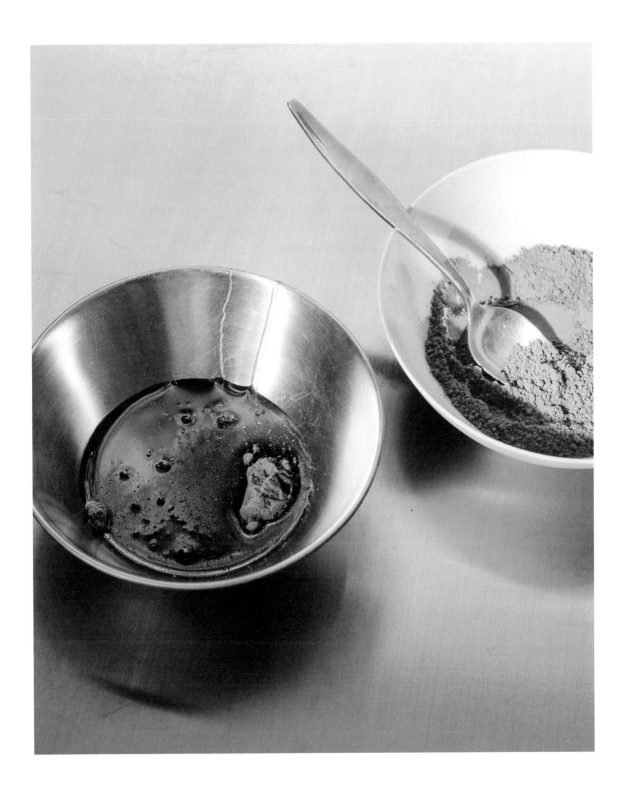

What Are Signs
of Stress in the Body?

Stress reveals itself in myriad ways—and it can be different for every person and change over time. As stress saps the parasympathetic nervous system, that over-exhaustion affects every major biological system in the body: primarily the endocrine, adrenal, digestive, respiratory, cardiovascular, nervous, and immune systems. So while stress affects the body universally, its symptoms will animate more locally:

BRAIN

Chronic stress deteriorates the mechanism of the brain responsible for concentrating and learning, forming memories, decision-making, judgment, social connection, making new brain cells, and controlling stress (cyclical, yes); and it can lead to issues like depression or diseases like Alzheimer's.

SPIRIT

Consistently activating the stress response is a mood killer and spiritual inhibitor. Excess cortisol in the brain and adrenal-fueled inflammation in the body are the main ingredients for things like anxiety, depression, irritability, feelings of disconnection, and loss of creative flow.

POWER

Our power, or our ability to rebound, recover, and reactivate, is directly affected by the stress response. An overabundance of stress hormones can stifle the function of immune cells, leaving you more vulnerable to infections and slowing the healing process. A body depleted of chi, prana, energy, or power is also one that experiences more fatigue, inflammation, pain, and decreased cardiovascular integrity.

SEX

All that's sexy, juicy, and divine takes a major hit from a frequently activated stress response. A stressed body is one that values survival, not procreation, much less pleasure and creativity. Stress affects sex on a number of levels: cortisol dampens the libido, makes orgasm difficult if not impossible, and throws off the menstrual cycle. Endorphins—which the body releases to mitigate pain during stress events—can block the release of hormones essential for making testosterone (our in-house Viagra), as well as for stimulating sperm and aiding the fertilization and implantation of eggs into the uterine wall. The rerouting of blood flow to more essential organs makes it harder to power up your pleasure centers.

BEAUTY

How we look on the outside is a direct reflection of our health on the inside. Stress dysregulates all of our physiological systems, and that adds up and prints out on the body as less lustrous and plump skin, accelerated aging, spots, acne or eczema outbreaks, puffiness, brittle nails, and thinning hair. High levels of cortisol can also prompt the body to store extra visceral or deep belly fat.

SLEEP

Stress unsettles the body and mind, creating a less-than-ideal environment for achieving deep rest. When in chronic stress you may have difficulty attaining deep rest needed for repairs and replenishment.

Stress + You

Part of this journey is figuring out what your unique stress response looks like. I'll give you a clue: It's subtle. Most people aren't handed a big, flashing sign that points to where and how stress is affecting their body. For many of us, it's what looks like an accelerated creep of aging—the gray hairs and fine lines appear faster, your jeans don't quite fit, you catch every flu going around, and you can barely muster the energy to do the things you once enjoyed. For others, it's conditions that we've been taught to accept as "normal"—allergies, digestive issues, skin conditions, inflammation-related discomfort, low libido, or a racing mind. In some cases, ignoring these seemingly benign acute symptoms will turn them into that big flashing sign that is now a chronic condition, i.e., heart disease, diabetes, arthritis, Alzheimer's. Luckily, we have the tools to help the body better cope, heal, and rebound so that we don't have to get to that place of crisis before doing something about it (though these same tools are certainly available for your support in moments of crisis, too). First, you need to change your expectations—expect better for yourself! Don't accept not thriving or not feeling great. Don't buy into the idea that your life-force will start dimming as you hit thirty-five. Your inner and outer wellness is essentially a printout of what has been happening inside your body up until this moment, and you've officially been handed the ability to hit "refresh" on the whole program.

We can't possibly hold the answers for how to completely eliminate stress from our lives (nor would we want to—as we'll explore in the next chapter). Instead, we can focus on how to fortify ourselves against the inevitable. This is where adaptogens come in.

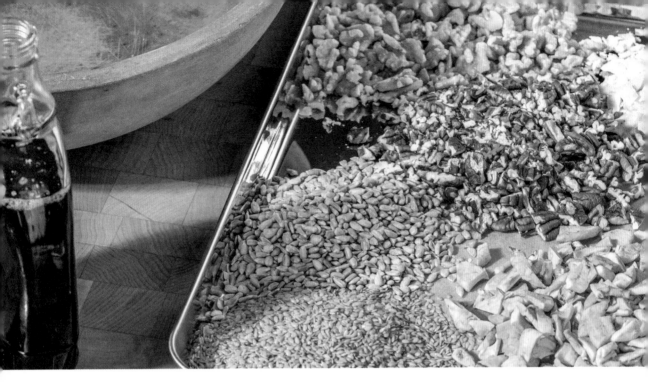

WHY A STRESSED GUT IS A STRESSED YOU

The gut is at the very center of your health. It's responsible for straightforward things like digestion and output (not particularly glamorous but essential for detoxification), but more surprisingly, it houses about 80 percent of our immune system mechanisms and is a direct link to the brain and our nervous system. The rich ecosystem of bacteria that resides there is responsible for keeping our bodies healthy by supporting the immune system, absorbing nutrients, keeping inflammation in check, and balancing hormones, while also promoting mood regulation and optimal brain function. And

these microscopic organisms are also to thank for helping us tune in to the very core of our being when we need a guiding light—quite literally trusting our gut.

Because the brain, gut, and immune system are inextricably linked, when the brain triggers a stress response, the gut is in on the action. And because the stress response is not without consequences on the body, these biochemical changes have a major and immediate effect on gut function—and, by extension, our overall health. When the body experiences chronic or prolonged stress episodes (every day), our bacteria friends

suffer. Cortisol is not gentle on the gut, and its assaults—decreased blood flow, increased permeability, and, in turn, increased presence of "bad" bacteria and unchecked inflammation—decrease the numbers and diversity of its flora. When that happens, you start to see things like irritable bowel syndrome, heartburn, exhaustion, nutritional deficits, mood disruption, less-than-ideal cognitive function, neurological maladies, sleep dysfunction, hormonal imbalance, skin and weight issues, and other signs of accelerated aging.

What Is an Adaptogen?

Simply put, adaptogens are plants. And these plants are products of their environment, thriving in some of the harshest climates on Earth. The high altitude, oxygen deprivation, extreme radiation from the sun, and punishing temperatures they've had to endure (some survived the Ice Age) are what make them so uniquely potent. It's that same adaptive energy that helps us gracefully keep up with the never ending and unexpected changes in life.

Though they have been used for centuries in traditional healing practices like Ayurveda and traditional Chinese medicine, the term "adaptogen" is neither ancient nor rooted in herbal medicine. It's a modern label that was first used in 1961 by research scientist Dr. I. I. Brekhman. As he concluded through scientific measure, adaptogens are nontoxic plants that help the body adapt to stress on a cellular level. They increase resistance to physical, biological, emotional, and environmental stressors; chemically support homeostasis; and regulate the body's systems.

In essence: If stress is dragging you down, adaptogens will boost you up. If stress drives you to the point of a fight-or-flight response, adaptogens will help you stay calm and collected. Adaptogens don't quash stress: rather, they promote the body's ability to cope with stress and recover from it by boosting the adaptive stores in every one of your biological systems. Ultimately, adaptogens have the power to restore the supply of life-force energy in the body, mind, and spirit.

Adaptogens work through two master control systems: the HPA axis (the hypothalamic-pituitary-adrenal axis, which controls endocrine, nervous system, and some immune function), and the SAS, or sympathoadrenal system, which is our fight-or-flight response. They have the power to:

1   Modulate the sensitivity of the hypothalamus so that less cortisol is secreted during the stress response.

2   Recharge the adrenal glands, helping them to return to a state of rest after a stress episode.

3   Prevent cortisol-induced mitochondrial dysfunction. Mitochondria are the "engines of our cells," and when they no longer function appropriately, this can contribute to conditions such as chronic fatigue syndrome and fibromyalgia. Adaptogens help keep the mitochondria properly functioning even when under chronic stress conditions.

4   Act as "immunomodulators"—they can fine-tune the immune system. If the immune system is sluggish, adaptogens enhance the immune response. If the immune system is overactive—for instance, with allergies or an autoimmune disorder—adaptogens help reregulate that response.

5   Are "amphoteric"—they balance the body's pH levels and minimize damaging inflammation.

6   Are "bidirectional"—they can either calm the activity of hyperfunctioning systems or strengthen the activity of low-functioning systems.

7   Are "nonspecific"—they adapt their function to your body's specific needs so that you can find your version of a healthy resting state.

Your Life on Adaptogens

Adaptogens help you feel your true potential and, perhaps most powerfully, they will give you the perspective to advocate for other types of simple self-care practices. Their effects may initially seem understated, but with habitual use their benefits prove to be real, powerful, and undeniable. A daily practice of taking adaptogens can do wonders for generally reviving the systems. While all adaptogens have a bidirectional effect on stress, each also has a distinct profile of qualities that shine on specific systems: Some slow the biology of aging, some come to the aid of a worn-out immune system, some sharpen the mind, and some charge physical performance. Some are more energizing, some are more calming, some are warming, some cooling, some moistening, and some drying. Homeostasis is always their end goal, but they arrive by a variety of paths. They have been shown to be capable of:

1   Preserving collagen protein for more elastic, radiant skin
2   Controlling stress-related weight gain
3   Reducing puffiness and taming inflammation
4   Curbing sugar cravings
5   Rebalancing sex hormones for stronger sex drive and virility
6   Regulating the gut and sustaining a vibrant microbiome
7   Slowing or reversing an aging process that has been accelerated

The benefits of adaptogens are both short and long term. If I'm having mental or general cognitive overload, I know I can make a tonic with some reishi or rhodiola and start to feel a shift in about twenty minutes. But I'm not just addressing a temporary situation; I'm proactively affecting my long-term health. I'm fending off the flu that my kid might bring home in the next month; I'm preventing the fritz-out that could occur on a Tuesday night; their amphoteric and immunomodulating properties help tame the inflammation, swelling, and other symptoms that arise from an autoimmune disorder; and, thanks to their neuroprotective power, I'm improving the plasticity in my brain and warding off degeneration that could eventually lead to Alzheimer's or dementia. These plants allow you to play preventative offense when it comes to your health, instead of reactionary defense. As aging is biological, not chronological, it's never too early or late to decide how you want to regenerate physically, emotionally, or mentally.

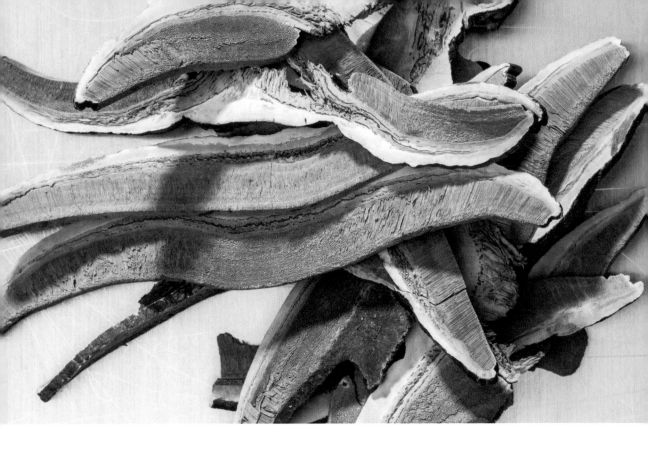

ANCIENT WISDOM AND MODERN INNOVATION

In Ayurveda, adaptogenic plants (or *rasayanas*) such as amla, ashwagandha, shatavari, and tulsi were believed to slow aging, revitalize the body, and ward off disease. This understanding had a strong influence on traditional Chinese medicine, as well as Tibetan and Islamic healing practices. The modern scientific study of adaptogens began in the 1940s, when Soviet scientists explored these plants for preventing and reducing illness, promoting homeostasis, and building strength. By the 1960s, Russian scientists were conducting hundreds of clinical studies on herbs used in Russian folk medicine. The studies measured the adaptogenic response of humans to stressful conditions such as heat, noise, exercise, and increased workload. They discovered improvements in hearing, mental alertness, work output, and athletic performance. These adaptogens were used by the Russian Olympic teams, and the athletes reported improved stamina, better performance, and shorter recovery times. By the 1970s, the Soviets had incorporated the adaptogens in their space program to help the cosmonauts' bodies better cope with the harsh conditions of interplanetary travel. Since then, Western researchers and scientists have observed how adaptogens regulate the hypothalamic, pituitary, adrenal access, HPA, and sympathoadrenal systems.

COMMUNAL

CARE

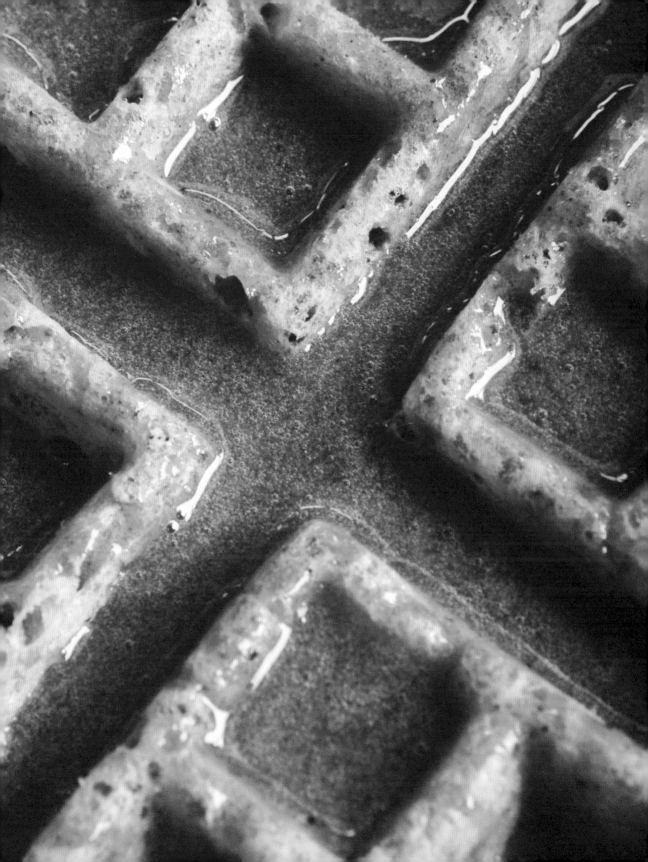

"Self-care" has gotten a bad rap as being selfish, but without advocating for our well-being we can't expect to show up for anyone or anything. Self-care is not a luxury item, and self-care is not an indulgence. It can be as free as a walk outside, as natural as prioritizing sleep, and as accessible as a hug. All support your immune system, sweeten your mood, and stoke energy. They, like adaptogens, reduce the effects of stress and sustain your overall quality of life. If you want to live in an expanded state and share that with the world, then making space for daily stress management will be your number one task—even if it's just choosing one adaptogen and having it in a cup of hot water once a day. It is not an extravagance; it's an essential, just like brushing your teeth! It's making the choice to properly equip and care for the one vessel that you're given to show up and do exactly what you came to do.

My goal is to help you find the most efficient, effective ways to help yourself; to connect you with the one or two (maybe three) things you can easily do each day that will deliver you to a more energized, productive, blissful place. The kind of healing that comes from your relationship with your body and your existing daily rhythm. Ultimately, the most powerful habit is the one you actually and consistently *do*.

The adaptogens you'll meet in this book are tools. They are each helpful in their own unique way, but you have to understand not just *how* to use them but also *when* you need them. That's where your innate knowledge of your body comes into play. One of the most important skills you can have is being able to tell when your adaptive energy is starting to run low. It's no different from looking at your phone to check your battery's status. If you're out and see that you only have 10 percent left, and you can't stop to charge, you know that you need to scale back on energy-draining behavior and be smart about what you use that energy for. You won't listen to music or read the news—you'll need to just keep your phone in your pocket in case you have to pull up a map or make an important call. You're going to be conservative until you can recharge. We all know how to take care of the energy in a phone or refuel a car—we have an ingrained understanding of what it means to see that little icon turn red. You need to attune to your body in this way. What is 100 percent for you? How do you feel when you're performing at your peak? What are the signs that energy is dwindling? Do you start to notice shifts in your body? Your mood? And what can you do that brings that energy back up? Now is the time to look at your own technological systems and think about how you can work with them efficiently.

It's important to believe that taking care of yourself doesn't mean you're weak. It's smart. I couldn't do half of the things that I do—run a company, have presence in my relationships, mother, and have energy for what the world asks for—if I didn't support my body's and spirit's needs. I'm not talking about radical life changes and time-consuming, esoteric habits; it's about small daily habits that bring us power, strength, intuition, intelligence, and resilience.

Don't Let Stress,
Stress You Out

Another misunderstanding about self-care is that the point is to eliminate all stress. So often I'm asked how I create balance or *avoid* stress. What I tell people is this: Don't let anyone sit there and tell you that in order to achieve the greatness they do—whether it's running a business or being

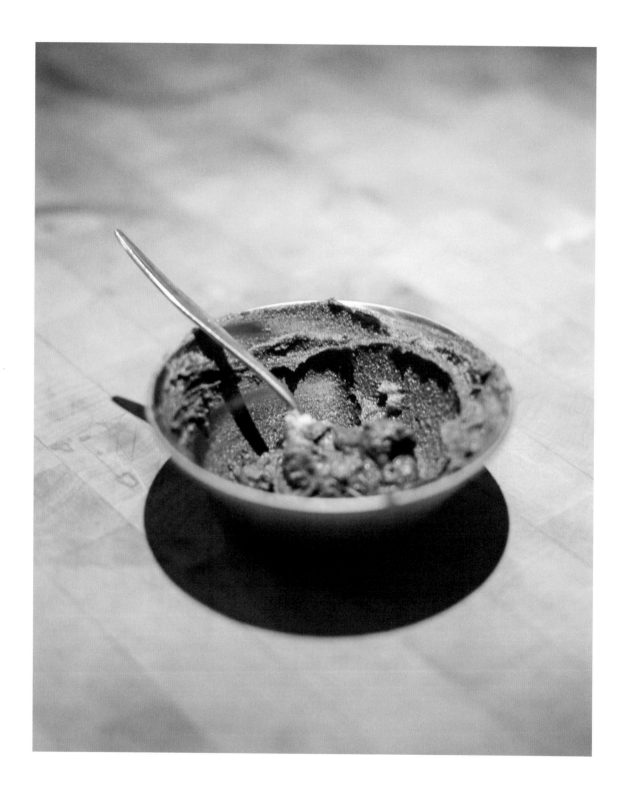

a full-time mom or both—that they just have some hot water and lemon in the morning, do some yoga, get a massage, have a little "me time," and then everything is amazing all the time. It's probably not true, and it's not something for you to compare yourself to. The reality is, we can't get rid of stress even if we try, so why continue to add stress by trying? The aim shouldn't be to control things like stress or aging or even disease, but rather, strengthening your vitality and intelligence through internal balance. If we maintain a strong immune system, healthy gut, and positive attitude, then we have the energy to react (or not react) very differently to triggers, including illness.

The key is to embrace the triggers, recognize the sources, and then protect and adapt. I'm not suggesting that you invite more stress into your life, but there are realities about living the lives we want to live, like not always getting enough sleep, too much screen time, and not fueling optimally every day, plus environmental factors that we have less control over. Also, some stress can be beneficial. It's a dynamic energy that drives and propels us forward. We actually *need* cortisol in order to function. When dosed in appropriate amounts, it's what motivates us to get out of bed in the morning, helps us power through the day, and recedes again at night to signal that it's time to sleep. Without it, we'd be listless, completely oblivious to our environment and potential threats.

So let's not fear stress. Instead, let's think about the different levels where we can meet it. At the most basic level, you can strengthen your somatic systems with adaptogens. When I feel overwhelmed by everything going on, and start to feel my endocrine and lymphatic systems out of balance, or know that I'm going into a period where I have a ton of work, lots going on at home, and travel, I think to myself, *That's a lot of energy, and it's ultimately going to help me move forward and accomplish things, but for now, it seems like a good idea to cut out social ambitions, rest where I can, meditate, get some walking in, and be sure to include adaptogens every day.*

You can live a long and healthy life in the face of stress, as long as you offer yourself support. It's really no different from wearing sunscreen. Like stress, some sun feels nice, even healthy. But you also know that too much can hurt. No one's thinking about how we're going to get rid of the sun or how we can all live in dark caves during the day. Instead, we accept the fact that if we're going to put ourselves directly in the sun's path, we're going to take appropriate measures. The same goes for stress: It's always going to be there, and if you're going to work and parent and get on airplanes and sleep less than you should for a month because that's who you are and what you want to do, then you need to protect yourself from getting burned. That's when you reach for the adaptogens.

I also believe that stress is a perception, and shifting that perception changes how we experience stress. One of the most stressed times in my life was when I was working for someone else, didn't have a child, and lived alone. I didn't have any responsibilities outside of showing up for my job. I remember one particular moment when I got a parking ticket outside of my house and I had a meltdown. A total world-is-ending meltdown. I'd burned through so much adaptive energy and was running on empty. Seeing a parking ticket felt like the end of my rope. It was like I had blinders on that made it hard to see how I could possibly have the time, capacity, or mental wherewithal to call an 800-number that's printed directly on the ticket and give them my credit card information. I can recall times when I've gone on vacation with nothing to do but relax and eat fruit and have still been stressed for some reason. Flash-forward to my life now, where I have more responsibility and much less free time to recharge, but I'm in my body and in tune with my energy, and the stress stays on the outside for the most part. I get to meet that bright sun with

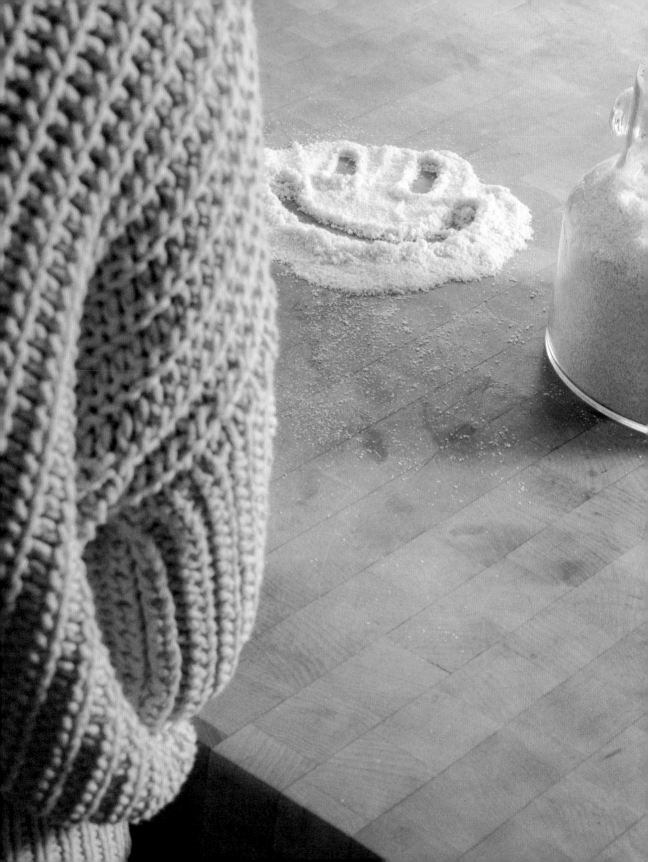

equal and opposite adaptive energy. That shift comes not only from the nutritive fortification of adaptogens and other simple self-care, but from perception. There's an epidemic of people walking around in constant overwhelm—we hear it all the time: "I'm just so busy and so stressed." Rather than saying, "I'm so stressed," you might instead say, "My battery is running low and I need to charge." No one would get mad at you if you had to jump off a call because your phone was about to die, and the world will not end if you need to stare out the window, or close your eyes, take some deep quality breaths, and have a few minutes to yourself. Doing these things every day keeps you from getting to the point where you feel like you can't get out from under the pressure; they give you the perspective to look back and realize maybe there was nothing to be so upset about after all.

Or even more radical, you could celebrate stress, reframing it altogether as something positive and growth inspiring. I love the way Dr. Pratima Richur puts it:

> No human being is immune to stress, but if we can change the perception of it, our physiological responses can also shift. Instead of being at the whim of stress, label it as a "challenge." This reorients you from a position of helplessness to empowerment. A challenge inspires a type of excitement, which, on the spectrum of emotions, is closer to happiness than sorrow. And re-labeling stress as something positive or solution-oriented provokes the secretion of a different set of hormones that actually benefit the body. Many people will attest to the fact that overcoming our challenges provides our greatest insights and growth. In this sense, reframing stress can facilitate in our potential to become fully realized souls.

All of these methods for meeting stress are meant to work with one another and should ideally be implemented *before* you get to the point of unconscious reaction. The preventative lifestyle is not a Spartan one. It doesn't require you to no longer celebrate, enjoy, and indulge. Instead, it asks that you adopt practices and forge relationships with supportive plants along the way. This is the road out of the unsustainable systems of our society and a gentle way back to the supportive embrace of life. The alchemy you will work with in this book supports the wisdom that already lives inside you and will lead you to some of your strongest allies, the adaptogens.

Your SPF
(Stress Protection Factor)

The journey you're about to embark on is one you can trace through human history on our evolutionary path toward higher efficiency and consciousness. Health issues that arise and call for your attention can be seen as pathways of transformation, or an escape from patterns that have been destructive. This revolution starts with tapping into your healer's intuition and embracing the intelligence of nature. We are all healers, and we all have the capacity to be healed—plants help to connect us to this energy. We're going to tap into your natural capacities and introduce you to a new circle of support. We're going to give you a potent new tool kit so that you can continue nurturing yourself and those around you.

It bears repeating that just because you're tuning in and taking off doesn't mean you now need ashram-level rituals. Rather than feeling like you need an entire kitchen of new foods, and a new pantry in order to get lifted on these adaptogens, hack your habits—plug into the daily rituals you already have. Because let's be real; you already have them: coffee or smoothies in the morning, a hit of chocolate in the afternoon, evening tea (or chocolate again), even just a bottle of water that you fill in the morning and sip on all day. Those are all opportunities to add adaptogens. These plants are perfectly happy to be swirled directly into coffee, tea, water, juice, milk, or smoothies. In chapter 10, you'll find recipes that are as easy to enjoy as they are to make. I wanted to think of more ways for you to plug them directly into the habits you already have while addressing the needs that will arise. I made them all doable and easy, requiring no special equipment or ingredients that you can't buy right off the Internet. Feel zonked at the office around 3:00 p.m.? Keep a jar of Brain Butter (page 137) in your desk drawer and eat a spoonful straight up. Take a love of ice cream and turn it toward Shatavari Fig Ice Cream (page 191) with a Shilajit Sex Drizzle (page 188). Swap your store-bought protein bars for Eleuthero Chocolate Chunk Cookies (page 168). (The Power recipes in particular are built to be especially portable for when you need to run, drive, or fly.) You can make big batches of Spiced Apple Reishi Granola (page 206), Horny Goat Weed Brownies (page 184), or Ashwagandha Cider Jellies (page 223). And if little by little you start feeling more adventurous and want to double- or triple-stack your adaptogens—Queen Healer Bread (page 149) slathered in Sex Honey (page 181) and Spirit Butter! (page 197)—these plants are happy to play.

This all comes back to the idea that the most powerful medicine is the one you take. These adaptogens can only give you their gifts if you invite them into your body. They don't care if they're tucked into pancake batter or chugged out of the milk jug. They just want to do right by you. So with that in mind, let's figure out which you'd like to summon in order to formulate your unique defense.

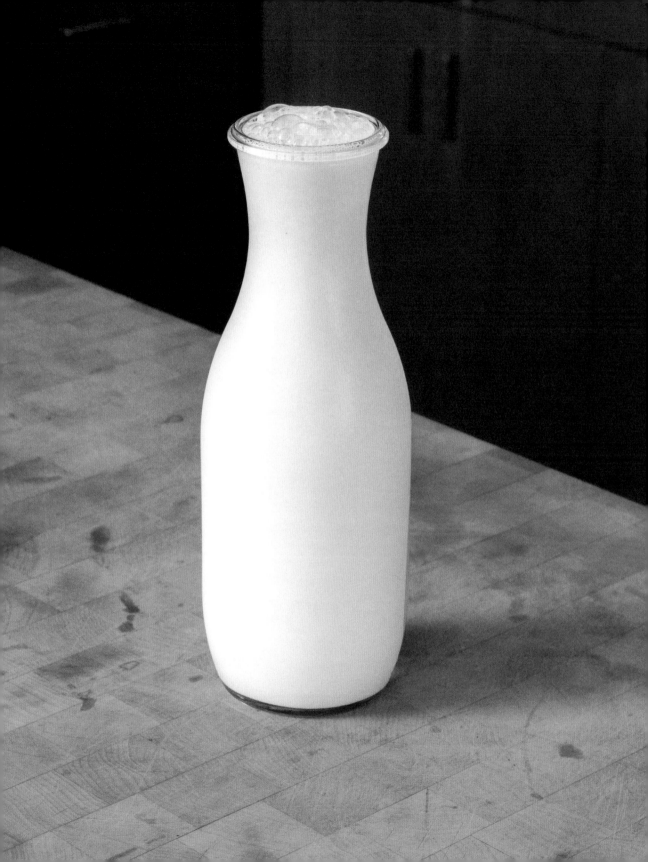

GLOSSARY

OF

ADAPTOGENS

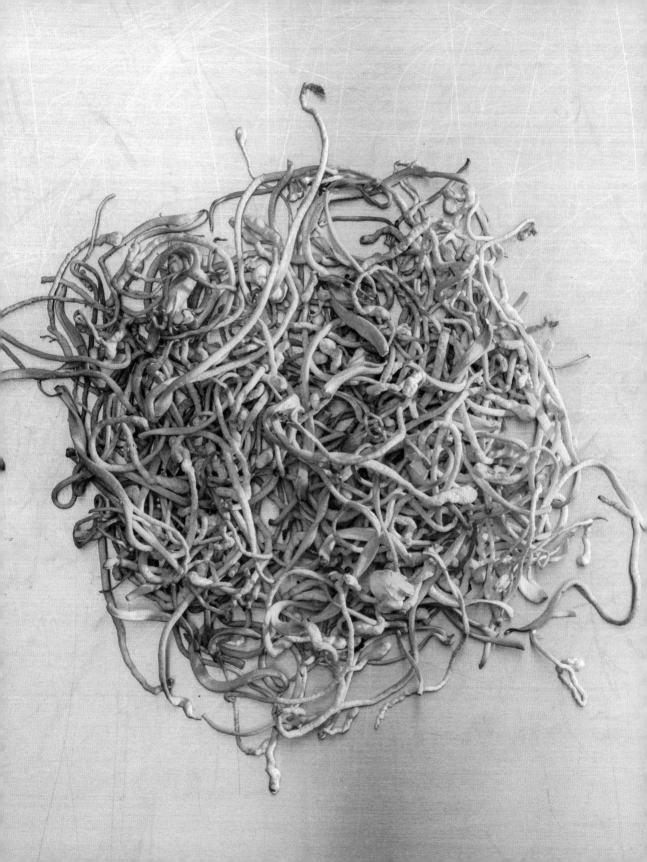

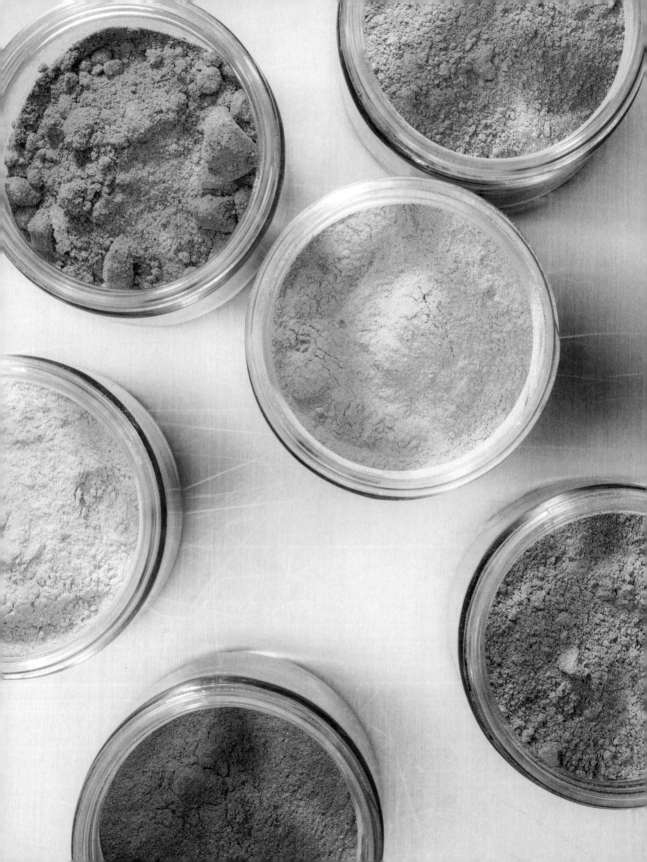

Welcome to your arsenal. These plants will be here for you in your moments of need. They will help you tune in and beam up, brightening your light when it feels dim, and connect you with your clearest, strongest, most radiant and resolved self. And if given the opportunity, each of these roots, leaves, and berries will continuously stand by you in good health and longevity.

In this chapter you'll find a glossary of all the adaptogens suggested throughout the book. You'll see that each has a primary application (or two) plus honorable mentions or secondary functions. It's a little bit like choosing a favorite child—they're all equally wonderful and powerful when it comes to whole body-mind healing, but they also have unique qualities that make them especially potent in different aspects of the body. The adaptogens' uses fall into six main categories: Beauty (skin, hair, and cellular health), Brain (memory, clarity of thought), Power (immunity, stamina, recovery), Spirit (mood, connectedness, creativity), Sex (intimacy, fertility, creativity), and Dream (rest, regeneration). Instead of jumping ahead to the chapters that interest you most, I invite you to spend some time with the adaptogens as they're described in this chapter. You'll begin to see the interconnectedness among them and their overlapping properties. As you tease out these patterns and relationships, you'll bring a deeper understanding of your apothecarial needs to the individual chapters.

To build your new adaptogenic tool kit, education is the first step. You have to take the time to try different plants and experience them. It's not required that you intellectualize each adaptogen; it may be enough to simply invite them into your body and feel what they have to offer you. A great way to start is to choose one to three plants that speak to you. Try one dose of each a day and continue for about a month. If you feel that's really working for you, keep going. If there are other adaptogens that have been calling to you, there's no harm in adding those or replacing others. It's amazing to me how differently the herbs speak to me, even from month to month. It makes sense, though—our needs are perpetually changing. And adaptogens are nimble enough to meet these nuanced fluctuations.

You may also want to ask yourself: Am I treating an *acute* situation or a *chronic* one (the result of an acute situation left untended—both of which are caused by stress)? Is this crisis or maintenance? In each chapter you'll find a description of what each looks like for that particular element of the body. For example: If you're having a spirit crisis, such as a surge of anxiety, then you'd refer to that chapter and find an adaptogen that sounds best for managing the condition. Then make sure you're enjoying two to three servings a day, every day, for thirty days. For maintenance, all the adaptogens are for you. Some days you may consider a double dose—if you feel a flu coming, you haven't gotten enough sleep, you're getting on an airplane—but for everyday wellness, see what you can weave into your existing daily rituals—coffee, smoothies, tea, granola—using the recipes. You'll be able to find more information about dosages and using the recipes as we focus on the individual adaptogens in the following chapters.

Bear in mind that nourishing and optimizing with adaptogens does not mean that you must abandon your medical practices and/or professionals. They do not contradict one another. This is a safe, effective path that is both interconnected and integrative (and much more affordable than critical care). If you are working with an acute or chronic condition, consult a functional medicine doctor or herbalist for guidance with regard to dosages and your exact medical history and for what may be appropriate for you.

If you'd like to read more about these adaptogens, where they come from, and how they work in the body, I highly recommend checking out *Adaptogens: Herbs for Strength, Stamina, and Stress Relief* by David Winston and Steven Maimes; and *Adaptogens in Medical Herbalism* by Donald R. Yance, CN, MH, RH(AHG).

WATCHING THE ADAPTOGENS AT WORK

While I am most comfortable deferring to the wisdom of herbalists, acupuncturists, and other traditional healers when it comes to addressing my own health, I am also a big believer in modern diagnostic tools, specifically blood tests, hormone panels, and microbiome analysis. They offer quantitative insight into your body and lend a numerical gauge for how your chosen mode of treatment is moving the needle. Having this information has allowed me to see, in black-and-white terms, how adaptogens have changed my biology over the course of addressing serious hormonal imbalances. If you're struggling with any kind of ongoing condition—trouble with fertility, exhaustion, thyroid issues, chronic disease—I strongly encourage you to create a touchstone for your health baseline with full blood, gut, and hormone panels. Then, in addition to riding the wave of feeling the adaptogens at work, you'll also be able to *see* them at work in your body and unpack those findings with your caregiver.

Tasting Notes and
Dosage Recommendations

The tasting notes and dosage recommendations included in this chapter are based on the highest-quality herbs and mushrooms that we source at Moon Juice. You may source herbs from wherever you like, but you may have to adjust your measurements and expectations accordingly. It is possible that the adaptogens you get elsewhere could be less effective, mixed with fillers, and untested for heavy metals or other contaminants. At Moon Juice, we shepherd the plant from crop to client using proprietary extraction methods that adhere to traditional practices and independent lab testing for potency and purity. This is not a sales pitch; it is my wanting to convey that selecting the best material is as important as remembering to take them daily.

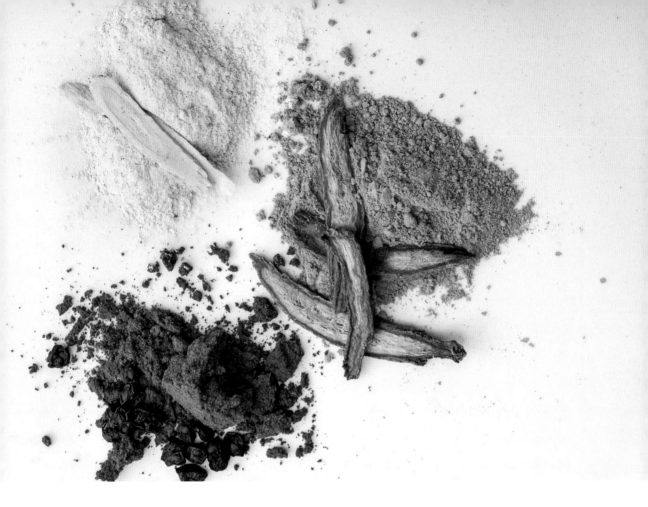

A NOTE ON DUSTS

Some of the most popular products that we sell at Moon Juice are our Dusts, or adaptogenic formulas that speak to a specific function: power, beauty, sex, spirit, dream, brain. The magic of these Dusts is that they are an efficient way to support the body—efficient in that a dose is one simple spoonful, and efficient in that the blend is already formulated. I find a place in my own practice for these Dusts and will readily recommend them to anyone seeking guidance for how to start an adaptogenic regimen or remedy a body in crisis. What I hope you'll find here is empowering information. You may use the called-for blends in each recipe or any Dust blend that you may have from Moon Juice.

Amla

Primary Benefit: Beauty
Honorable Mentions: Power, Spirit

Tasting Notes: A light powder that sits tannic on the tongue with a very tart flavor and subtle hints of tropical fruitiness. Pairs well with tropical fruit, citrus, berries, green smoothies, and ginger.

Amla, or Indian gooseberry, has been used in Ayurvedic healing, and its small, thorny trees are regarded as a sacred tree in native India. The fruit is dried and ground and has a combination of bitter, sour, and astringent tastes, pairing well with berries and fruit. It is worshipped because the fruits are both nourishing and believed to stimulate spiritual purity. It is a great stress-reliever that is known to soothe both muscles and mind, imparting feelings of peace. Amla is also one of the greatest protectors for the skin, defending against accelerated aging.

A rich source of vitamin C, amla is an antioxidant and anti-inflammatory, and it regulates blood sugar—essential keys to creating a foundation of wellness. Traditionally used for general care for the respiratory system, amla improves lung capacity and oxygen intake. It also facilitates production function of the liver, which is not only excellent for detoxification of the entire body but also crucial to the endocrine system and hormonal balance. It supports the immune system and increases vitality and stamina.

Ashwagandha

Primary Benefits: Spirit and Dream
Honorable Mentions: Brain, Power

Tasting Notes: A light and crystalline powder that has an intense, bitter, molasses-like flavor. It's both syrupy sweet and earthy bitter, with a little spice on the back of the tongue. Pairs well with chocolate, coffee, maple, and baked goods.

Ashwagandha is the potent flowering shrub that is relied upon heavily in Ayurveda to harmonize mind, body, and spirit. It's a calming, mineral-dense nervine that nourishes both the adrenal and thyroid glands to tame anxiety, renew vigor, and restore centeredness. Ashwagandha's antioxidant-rich properties are superior support for the immune system. It has been shown to lower blood sugar levels, reduce inflammation, and fight free radicals—all of which protect the brain from degeneration, improve memory, and prevent depression. It improves sleep and bumps virility. There will be variation in ashwagandha's appearance and flavor depending on what type of extraction method is used. I use one that is a dark, rich brown and has a candied nut smell and a heady, bitter malt taste. It pairs well with coffee, chocolate, milks, and caramel flavors.

Astragalus

Primary Benefit: Power
Honorable Mentions: Spirit, Brain

Tasting Notes: A rich brown dense and crystalline powder that has an intense, bitter molasses-like flavor. It's both syrupy sweet and earthy bitter, with a little spice on the back of the tongue. Pairs well with chocolate, coffee, maple, and baked goods.

Native to parts of the Middle East, as well as Korea and Mongolia, the roots of this flowering plant have long been prescribed by traditional Chinese medicine to fight off emotional stress and disease. It is used to calm nerves, regulate the adrenals, soothe inflammation, and increase circulation, which has a particularly potent effect on brain health. In fact, it has been used specifically to reinvigorate blood flow to the brain in the wake of a stroke. A daily ritual of this adaptogen becomes a protective shield around the brain to keep disease and mental stress out and nourishing, oxygenating blood in.

Astragalus houses three types of active compounds that lend their health-giving properties: saponins, flavonoids, and polysaccharides.[1] Saponins are thought to lower cholesterol, strengthen the immune system, and even prevent cancer;[2] antioxidant flavonoids fight free-radical damage, which can help prevent heart disease, cancer, and immunodeficiency viruses;[3] and polysaccharides are considered to have antimicrobial, antiviral, and anti-inflammatory properties.[4] Astragalus also contains unique compounds called "astragalosides," which wield the special adaptogenic power to bring the body toward equilibrium. This root is particularly beneficial for supporting the immune system,[5] helping the body heal more quickly, as well as to treat conditions such as asthma, rheumatoid arthritis, and allergies. It is considered to strengthen muscle tissue, tendons, ligaments, and lungs, as well as have an overall invigorating effect on the body. It's a multiuse adaptogen that can be called upon to quell infections and viruses,[6] beat back disease-causing inflammation,[7] protect the cardiovascular system,[8] regulate or prevent diabetes,[9] and support the renal system.[10]

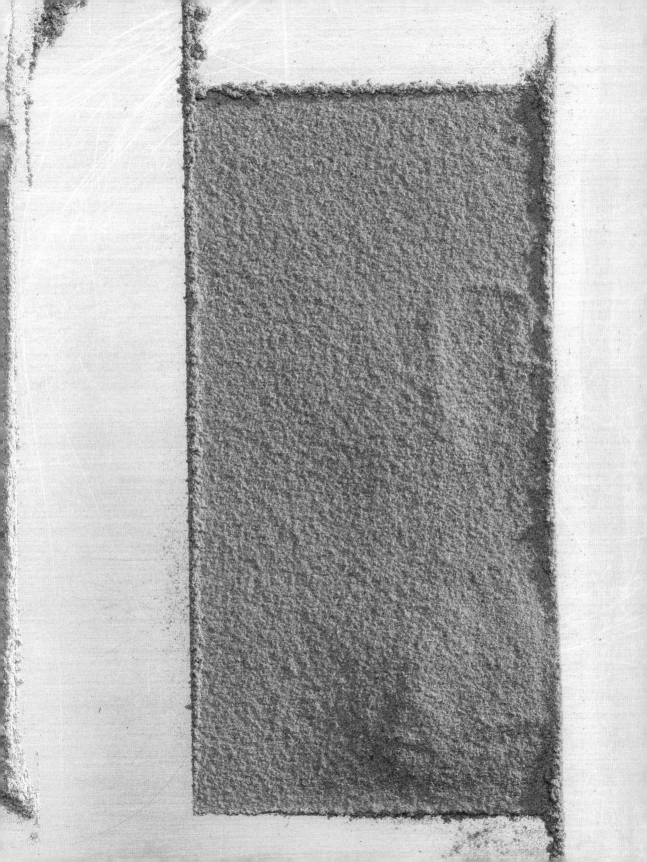

Cordyceps

Primary Benefit: Power
Honorable Mentions: Spirit, Sex

Tasting Notes: A golden powder with a slightly sweet anise-y, woody flavor. Pairs well with tropical fruits, citrus, ginger, chocolate, and coffee.

Cordyceps were traditionally gathered from the Himalayas in Bhutan and Tibet, as a fungus growing out of a caterpillar. In traditional Chinese medicine, the mushroom and the worm were used together, but this method is now rare, and most cordyceps mushrooms are cultivated without the worm, dried in the sun, and then ground into powder. Cordyceps survive in one of the harshest environments on Earth. Forced to adapt to high altitudes, lower oxygen levels, and freezing temperatures, these small, very rare mushrooms evolved to thrive, making them one of the most potent plant medicines today. In 1993, the Chinese women's Olympic track and field team broke multiple world records thanks to their cordyceps use. They were even tested for doping, but they were in fact shrooming. Cordyceps work to increase energy and endurance for athletes, encourage lung health and capacity, protect the liver and kidneys, help with age-related decline, and support the immune system.

Cordyceps balance the neuroendocrine system, in turn balancing and elevating mood. They are also great energizers, getting the brain clear and focused.

Cordyceps are known to be the sexiest of mushrooms, increasing libido and fertility in both men and women. Known as the "Himalayan Viagra," the Tibetans already downloaded what science now proves. The pharmacological and biological constituents of cordyceps bump energy, stamina, endurance, and recovery, so these Himalayan wonders will get the juices flowing, prevent impotence, encourage fertility, and enhance the libido.

Eleuthero

Primary Benefit: Power
Honorable Mentions: Brain, Spirit

Tasting Notes: A blond powder with a mild woody, smoky taste—almost like palo santo. Pairs well with vanilla, milks, fruit, caramel, and nuts. It also pairs nicely with chocolate and coffee, though it's not begging to be masked by those flavors.

Eleuthero, also known as Siberian ginseng, comes from a low shrub native to the high mountains of Siberia, China, Korea, and Japan. Its root, stem, and bark have all been used in traditional Chinese medicine and Ayurveda for centuries, as well as by Russian Olympians in the 1960s and '70s. It's wonderful for immunity, stamina, athletic performance, and brain function while working under stressful conditions. This plant is best for the constant traveler and those who press on despite knowing they haven't slept or rested enough. Not only will it power your day, but it will also aid in a solid night's sleep—when you actually do get to rest. Eleuthero is the ultimate jet lag, no sleep, physical recovery, flu season, and overworked brain remedy.

A proven mood elevator, eleuthero lowers cortisol levels, reduces stress, and discourages depression. And by supporting the circulatory system, eleuthero fosters focus and keeps the mind sharp. It also can help encourage healthy brain cell function.

Epimedium

Primary Benefit: Sex
Honorable Mentions: Power, Brain

Tasting Notes: A rich brown powder with a sweet caramel-like aroma and a light café con leche flavor with slight astringency. Plays well with baked goods, milks, vanilla, nutty malted flavors, honey, maple, chocolate, coffee, and dark berries.

Epimedium, also known as horny goat weed, is a flowering plant that is wild harvested in its native Asia and the Mediterranean. Epimedium has been used for thousands of years in traditional medicines and folk remedies because of its powerful anti-inflammatory and immune-strengthening properties, as well as its potent antiaging effects on the body. It is the most powerful plant on the planet for erectile dysfunction and boosts both male and female libido. Promoting testosterone production, this adaptogen has long been used by athletes to improve endurance and stamina. Like the vigor and passion it produces in the bedroom, epimedium can prepare the body for physical activity and exercise. It is a multiuse remedy that works from within to tame inflammation, get the blood flowing, and ignite an inner spark. Epimedium gets juices flowing in the brain as well as the body, stimulating cell growth, nerve activity, and circulation to the brain, and improving memory, focus, and learning ability. A powerful antioxidant, it also preserves nerve health.

Ginseng

Primary Benefit: Brain
Honorable Mentions: Sex, Power

Tasting Notes: A rich brown powder with an intense, mushroom-y, earthy aroma and a bitter, slightly astringent flavor. Pairs best with chocolate, coffee, and maple. It's also a great addition to savory dishes like soups and lentils.

Ginseng, used in traditional Chinese medicine and native to China and Korea, is now extremely difficult to source in the wild, but it originally grew in the mountainous forests. Its potency lies in its supreme ability to energize; it is particularly nourishing to the adrenals, kidneys, and immune system. Ginseng is soothing to inflammation and allergies, balancing to hormones, particularly nourishing to those with chronic or adrenal fatigue, and also restorative to those who are so depleted that they are unable to sleep.

Ginseng is known for its effect on male and female libido. Used to treat impotence, encourage arousal, and boost testosterone, Ginseng is a proven natural aphrodisiac. By working on the central nervous system, it encourages both sex hormones and sexual fluids.

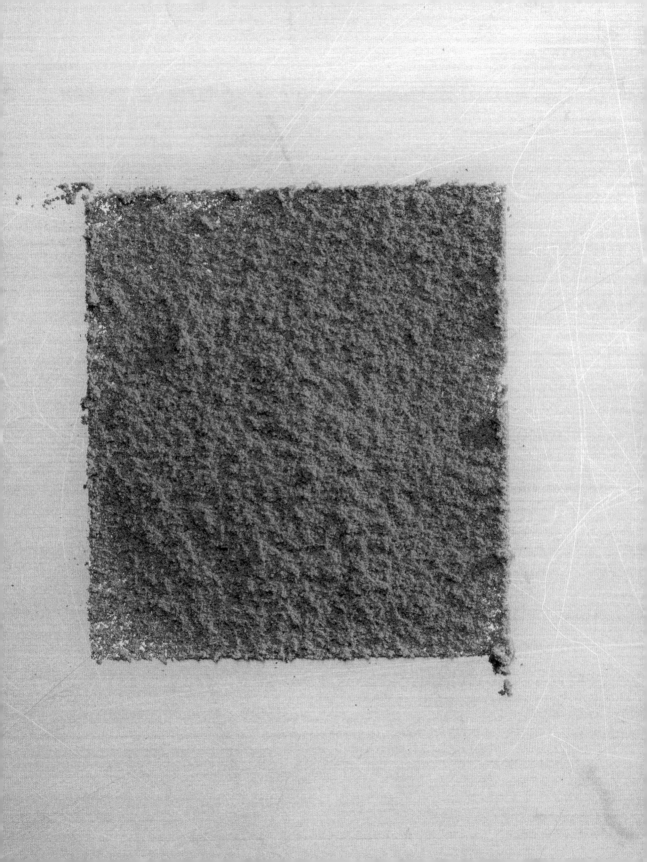

Licorice

Primary Benefit: Dream
Honorable Mentions: Spirit, Power

Tasting Notes: A blond powder with a sweet, licorice-like aroma and a bright, astringent bitterness. This is one for pairing with chocolates, coffees, and dark honeys, which help integrate the bold flavor.

Licorice or "sweet root," hailing from Europe, Asia, and North America, was used by ancient Romans and Greeks, Ayurveda, and traditional Chinese medicine. By the twentieth century, its curiously sweet flavor turned it into a popular candy, with fewer people recognizing its adaptogenic properties. Licorice regulates the endocrine system and is strengthening to metabolic function and immunity. Licorice also balances the adrenal system, which can help energize, alleviate chronic fatigue, and help with post-workout recovery. Taken after a workout, it helps reduce muscle pain and soreness. Licorice is a powerful relaxant when taken in the evening. Particularly supportive to female hormone balance, it can be used for PMS and the discomforts of both menstruation and menopause. Containing various antidepressant compounds and hormone-regulating abilities, licorice is an effective way to lift the spirit.

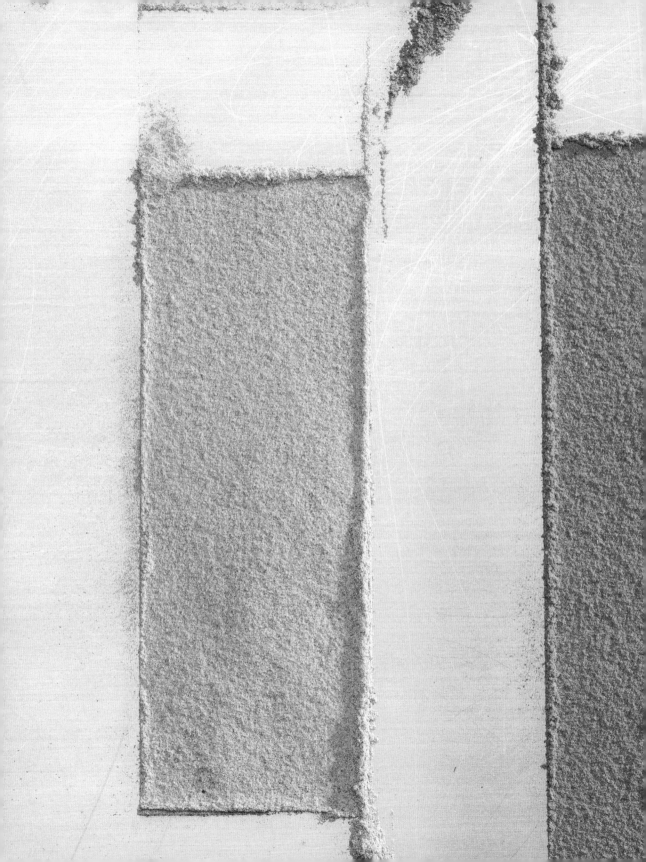

Mucuna

Primary Benefit: Spirit
Honorable Mentions: Brain, Sex

Tasting Notes: A rich brown powder with a sweet caramel-like aroma and a light café con leche flavor with slight astringency. Plays well with baked goods, milks, vanilla, nutty malted flavors, honey, maple, chocolate, coffee, and dark berries.

Mucuna, used in Ayurveda, traditional Chinese medicine, and shamanic medicine, is native to tropical areas of Africa and Asia. Mucuna is a potent psychoactive. Its natural bounty of L-dopa—an amino acid and hormone that is a precursor for neurotransmitters such as dopamine, epinephrine, and norepinephrine—supplies the brain with the fuel to create more of the beneficial neurotransmitters dopamine, epinephrine, and norepinephrine. As a result, mucuna supports all-around brain health. It combats symptoms of depression, increases focus, and curbs memory loss. It has even been used as a natural treatment for Parkinson's disease, a progressive nervous system disorder caused by the decrease of dopamine in the brain. Mucuna also serves as a potent aphrodisiac. It arouses libido in both sexes, heightening the senses and igniting desire. Mucuna also stimulates testosterone production in men and wards off menstrual cramps in women. Able to nourish and revitalize the whole body, it supports mental and physical health with both invigorating and calming effects.

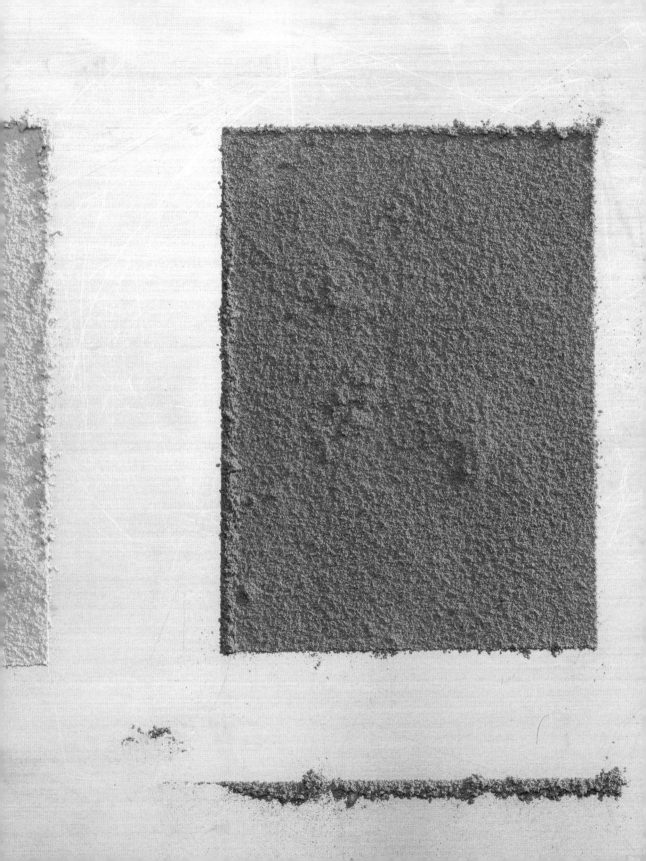

Reishi

Primary Benefits: Brain, Sleep, and Spirit
Honorable Mention: Power

Tasting Notes: A dark brown powder with a strong, botanical aroma and an intensely tannic taste with some bitterness. Pairs well with chocolate and coffee.

This mushroom grows on trees in the United States, Asia, and even parts of the Amazon, under a wide range of conditions. Reishi has been crowned queen healer by traditional Chinese herbalists for centuries because of its ability to strengthen the heart and mind, allowing you to unlock creativity and connect. This super mushroom is a brain nourisher, immune supporter, energizer, stress reliever, and beauty food. It has neuroprotective qualities, which not only help dissipate stress-induced brain fog and enhance memory but also are also highly therapeutic for neurodegenerative disorders, as reishi supports the production of nerve growth factor (NGF). Reishi improves adrenal and pituitary function and is packed with antioxidants, which strengthen the body's resistance to disease and infection. It stabilizes the nervous and digestive systems, reduces inflammation, balances hormones, supports reproductive health, and regulates the thyroid.

Rhodiola

Primary Benefit: Brain
Honorable Mentions: Spirit, Power

Tasting Notes: A light, pillowy powder with no aroma, a mild vegetal sweetness, and a slight bitter aftertaste. Pairs well with milks, vanilla, baked goods, maple, honey, date, banana, coffee, and chocolate.

Rhodiola has been used in traditional Chinese medicine and grows at some of the highest altitudes on Earth. This hardy plant can be found in the Arctic areas of Eastern Europe and Asia. In its native environment, rhodiola has managed to adapt to some of the world's harshest conditions such as extreme temperatures and sun exposure. The result is an adaptogen with an amazing power-up effect on humans. Rhodiola helped early Sherpas as they climbed Mount Everest; the Vikings and ancient Greeks looked to it for strength; and early Russian herbalists prescribed it as a remedy for depression. It sustains endurance, fights fatigue, and increases cardiovascular function and lung capacity while also easing stress and lifting moods. Another incredible feat of this adaptogen is its ability to help your body burn fat. Rhodiola contains rosavin, a natural trigger that signals the body to burn fat while soothing and toning muscles. Rhodiola increases athletic stamina and recovery, as it works on hormonal harmony by balancing the endocrine system. An ancient remedy for anxiety and schizophrenia, rhodiola is prescribed today as a natural antidepressant. By lowering levels of cortisol, rhodiola pulls the body out of fight-or-flight mode and keeps everyday stress at bay.

Schisandra

Primary Benefit: Beauty
Honorable Mentions: Brain, Power, Spirit

Tasting Notes: A vibrant deep berry, rust-colored powder with some moisture to it. Treasured as the five-flavored berry, schisandra truly does encapsulate all five flavors: sweet, sour, bitter, salty, and pungent. It is extremely potent. It is fun to rest a pinch on your tongue and have a little party in your mouth, in the way you might a Szechuan peppercorn or a peppermint. Schisandra pairs well with citrus (especially grapefruit), berries (especially strawberries), iced teas, green smoothies, and dark chocolate.

Native to the harshest climates of China, schisandra is a red berry found on vines. Taoist monks often used schisandra in ceremonies and during prayer. Prized in traditional Chinese medicine as a longevity and beauty berry, this antioxidant-rich tonic repairs the cell and tissue damage that speed up the aging process while improving skin and liver health by nourishing from within. It supports the endocrine system, strengthens the immune system, and gently energizes the nervous system while taming anxiety and supporting reproductive health, fertility, virility, and libido. Schisandra has been used as a supplement for athletic training because of its ability to enhance endurance, stamina, and performance. By regulating and reducing stress hormones in the blood, schisandra also works well to mellow and clear the mind. As a true spirit lifter, the berry can be used for enhancing a meditation practice. Schisandra also assists with fine-tuning the brain, offering mental clarity and focus. It has been used for centuries in traditional Chinese medicine to help increase concentration, motivation, and memory. It has also been shown to protect against a number of common neurological disorders, such as depression and anxiety.

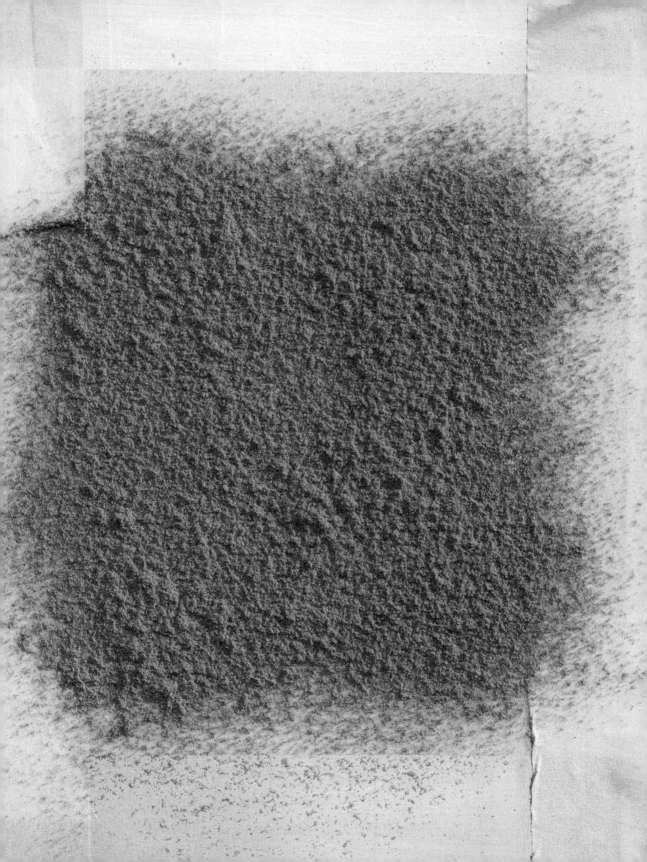

Shatavari

Primary Benefit: Sex
Honorable Mentions: Beauty, Power

Tasting Notes: A light, pillowy powder with no aroma and a mild vegetal sweetness with a slight bitter aftertaste. Pairs well with milks, vanilla, baked goods, maple, honey, date, banana, coffee, and chocolate.

Used in Ayurveda and grown throughout Nepal, India, and Sri Lanka, this powerful plant from the asparagus family is harvested for its thick, succulent roots. Shatavari simultaneously calms and energizes. It's a powerful aphrodisiac and primarily used to support sexual health. It has been called "the female Viagra." Shatavari will pick you up, dial you in, and turn you on. It is considered the "queen of herbs" for its effect on female sexual health. *Shatavari* literally translates to "she who has one hundred husbands," and in Ayurveda it is considered the ultimate women's tonic, supporting through each phase of life. But it is also just as appropriate in tonics for men, as it increases testosterone, semen count, and arousal. Shatavari literally gets the juices flowing—it coats and soothes mucus membranes, restoring moisture in tissues from the yoni to the face. Shatavari brings hormonal harmony, which in turn supports a healthy reproductive system, strengthening the uterus and promoting breast milk production. It can relieve cramps; regulate menstruation; optimize fertility; and alleviate menopausal symptoms like night sweats, mood swings, and hot flashes, while also promoting the same fertile glow that women enjoy in pregnancy. This adaptogen is also a strong anti-inflammatory that contributes to radiant skin and healthy hair.

Shilajit

Primary Benefit: Sex
Honorable Mentions: Brain, Power

Tasting Notes: A very dark resin or powder with a funky aroma and a potent smoky flavor. Pairs well with dark chocolate and coffee.

Referred to as "conqueror of mountains and destroyer of weakness" in Sanskrit, shilajit has been used as a traditional remedy for over five thousand years in Ayurveda and traditional Chinese medicine. Shilajit is an ancient tar-like substance that contains over eighty-five minerals and trace elements that the body needs to function at its peak. Native to the Tibetan and Himalayan mountains, shilajit is found deep in rock crevices and ranges from dark brown to black in color. After seeing monkeys eating it, Tibetans believed it would help instill strength and power in humans. They weren't wrong. Shilajit energizes by working with the body's mitochondria to convert oxygen and nutrients into raw physical power. It revitalizes the body, sparking libido, boosting fertility, enhancing athletic performance, and fighting chronic fatigue. Shilajit also promotes brain health, nurturing cells and circulation. Rich in fulvic acid, considered to be one of the most chemically active and nutrient-rich compounds found in soil, this curative matter has been shown to fend off age-related cognitive impairment, has been prescribed for brain trauma to promote healing, and is used as a treatment for mild cases of Alzheimer's. Shilajit is also packed with B-complex vitamins and as such has been used to treat symptoms of epilepsy. And its ability to balance GABA (gamma-aminobutyric acid) means that shilajit can help soothe seizures and improve overall focus and memory functions.

Tulsi

Primary Benefit: Beauty
Honorable Mentions: Spirit, Power, Brain

Tasting Notes: A green powder with strong notes of dried cut grass and a mellow, salty, and bitter taste. Pairs well with fruit, green smoothies, and herbal salad dressings.

Tulsi is an herb native to India. Considered a sacred plant by Ayurveda, it's also known as holy basil. It's an ancient remedy for soothing body and mind, alleviating depression, and regulating hormones. It promotes circulation, normalizes blood pressure, controls blood sugar, reduces cortisol, and soothes the respiratory and digestive systems. It aids against stress-related weight gain, helps with bloating, and nourishes the blood by detoxifying it, making it a potent remedy for acne and eczema. It's also rich in antioxidants, which protect the skin from oxidative damage and signs of aging.

DR. MAYA SHETREAT-KLEIN
ON ADAPTOGENS FOR PREGNANCY AND KIDS

Can you take adaptogens if you're pregnant?

Adaptogens can offer wonderfully gentle and supportive nourishment during your pregnancy. Making sure your health-care practitioner is comfortable with your taking them, these plants in particular offer abundant prenatal support: amla, reishi, shatavari.

Can I give adaptogenic herbs to my child? How do these herbs benefit children specifically?

Yes, there are several adaptogenic herbs that can be wonderful for children. Because children face inevitable physical and emotional challenges over their childhood—which is normal and actually good (to a degree)—they can benefit tremendously from the balance offered by adaptogenic herbs. In addition, the rapid changes in their physiology during these critical windows of development render them vulnerable, and adaptogenic herbs can help them to be more resilient.

Plants are as complex as we are, so the effects are varied and far-reaching. Sometimes the promises can sound too good to be true, but both the scientific literature and hundreds of years of recorded use support these benefits.

What are your favorite herbs for children?

I love tulsi for its gentle, calming effect. Tulsi has antiviral, antibacterial, and antifungal properties while simultaneously supporting the immune system, which makes it great for kids who need that extra boost to their immunity. It protects against cancer as well as toxic exposures by boosting the cells' natural detoxification mechanisms, especially in the liver. Tulsi also balances blood sugar levels, for those kids who have lots of highs and lows in their energy around their mealtimes. Ashwagandha is another wonderful and balancing adaptogen for children that I frequently recommend in my practice. It is useful for

increasing calm, improving sleep, boosting thyroid function, fighting cancer, balancing immune function, and enhancing focus. I also love medicinal mushrooms like reishi, which support mitochondrial health—so that these incredible energy makers of the cells function more optimally. This means that you'll see better brain function and energy, which can be helpful to every child, from the extra-fatigued kid to the athlete. They also balance the immune system, reducing allergic response so you'll see fewer allergies and less asthma, while at the same time boosting the nonspecific immune system to fight colds, flus, and other infections.

Are there dosage guidelines?

Start low and go slow. Adaptogens can work quickly, but the shifts can also be gradual. One is not better than the other, but it can take time to get a real sense of the improvements. Remember that with kids (and most people), less is more.

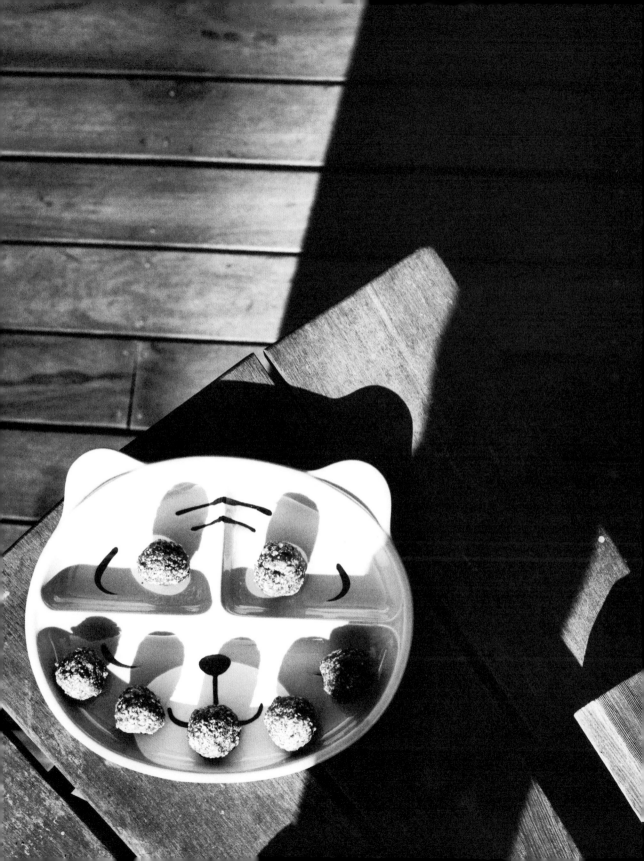

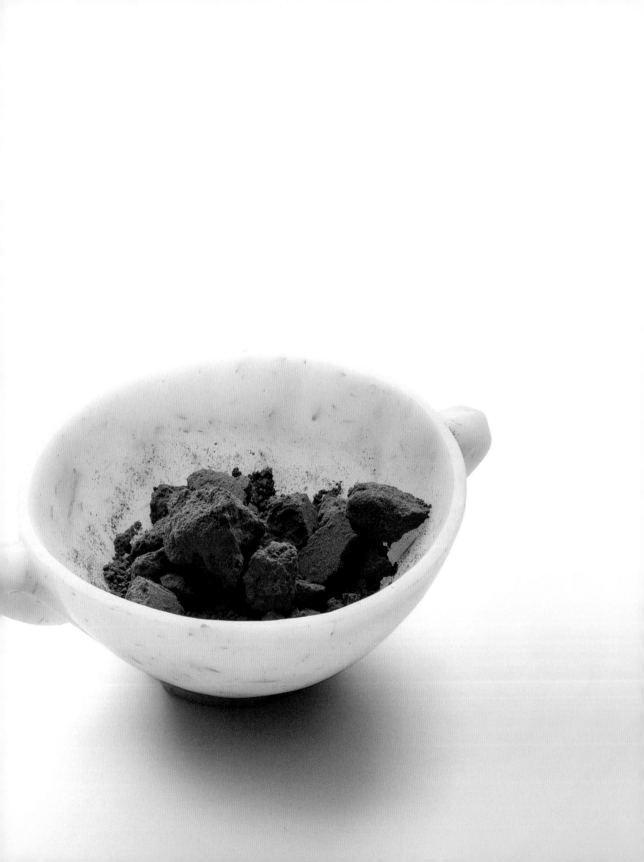

DOSES

Herb	MIN. PER DAY		MAX. PER DAY	
	tsp	gm	tsp	gm
Amla	⅛	.5	⅓	1
Ashwagandha	⅛	.3	½	1
Astragalus	1	2.25	2	4.5
Cordyceps	1	1	3	3
Eleuthero	1	2	2	4.5
Epimedium	1/16	.2	⅓	1
Ginseng	¼	1	¾	3
Licorice	⅛	.3	1	1.6
Mucuna (10% L-dopa)	1/12	.23	⅓	1
Reishi	1	1	4	4
Rhodiola	1/16	.15	⅛	.34
Schisandra	1	1	2	2
Shatavari	⅛	.4	¼	.8
Shilajit	1/16	.22	¼	1
Tulsi	½	1.5	1	3

SPIKE

YOUR DIET

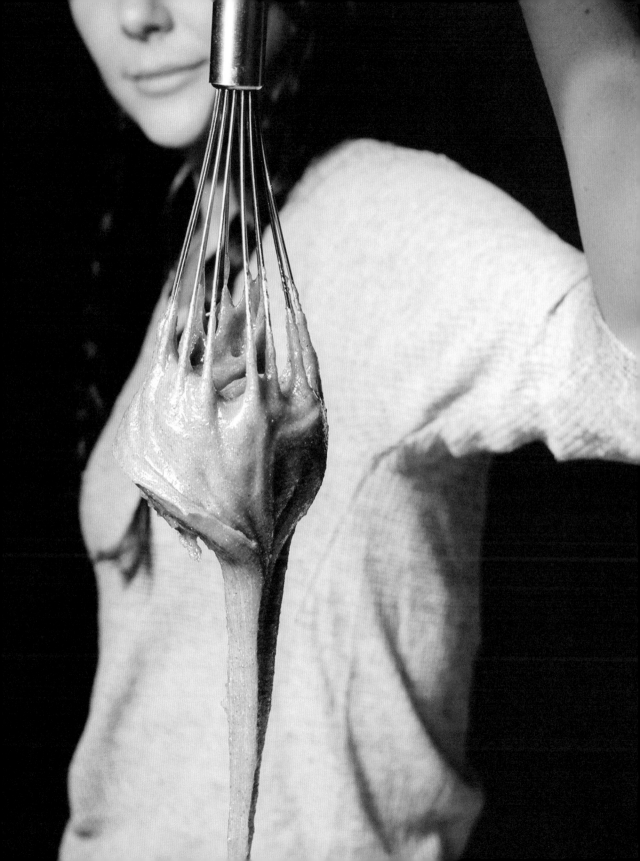

Included in each of the following chapters are recipes for "functional foods," foods that work *with* your body, not *against* them, and foods that go beyond satiation. These are items you can make in large batches and store so they're ready when you're hungry (pancake mix, brownie mix, granola), things you can keep in your freezer and eat as is or blended into smoothies, and adaptogen-infused honeys and butters that become instant tonics when blended with hot water, spread on toast, or eaten off the spoon, between meetings, during physical practices, or in the car. Invite these plants into your kitchen, your meals, and your snacks. With this type of repletion, you will find ease in the healing from the plants, as well as a natural alliance and understanding.

You'll also *enjoy* these recipes. My love of food is far too strong to suggest anything that won't bring pleasure along with the healing. Each adaptogen has its own poetic flavor, from earthy cordyceps and reishi, which play so nicely with cacao and cinnamon, to anise-y ginseng and spiced schisandra. Tasting the adaptogens is a powerful therapeutic tool, one that's at the foundation of Ayurveda and is considered in the curative effect on body, mind, and spirit. Each taste has its own emotional and energetic properties, and it's through the experience of flavor that we can truly harness a plant's healing potential, as well as cultivate a deeper relationship with it.

As you move through these recipes, consider them not just a vehicle for the adaptogens but also an opportunity to savor the plants. It's no different from drinking a glass of wine and teasing out each note and element of terroir—or beer, tea, coffee, and dark chocolate. At first those things may taste bitter, funky, or earthy, but once you know where that plant was from and how it was prepared it becomes a joy and art in your life. These adaptogens are no different. Once you begin to get into the rhythm, there's no going back. These plants are too effective to ignore once you've experienced them.

Stack
Your Habits

These recipes have been calibrated to speak to the specific chapters in this book: "Beauty," "Brain," "Power," "Sex," "Spirit," and "Dream." In each chapter, you'll find a signature dry-mix herbal blend, infused butter (coconut or ghee), and honey. These are your most basic building blocks. The dry mixes are great for traveling and adding to water, tea, or smoothies (or stored in veggie capsules and taken as part of your supplement regiment). Kept in an airtight container, the adaptogens will stay potent for up to a year. The infused butters and honeys can be eaten off the spoon; or spread onto toast; or—my favorite mode of transportation—blended into daily tonics (recipes for which I've also included in each section). I consider these honeys, butters, and tonics to be your adaptogenic staples because the honeys and butters are easy to make in big batches and will be shelf-stable for up to a year if you're mindful of simple sanitary practices, like not double-dipping. I love having these tools at the ready because they're an easy, joyful way of taking your medicine, particularly when you don't have time to make a meal or snack. (They also make a lovely gift.) Infused honeys and butters can be a great way of addressing more than one area of focus at once. For example, if you're working on brain chemistry and mood, you could make a batch of Brain Honey (page 137) and

Spirit Butter (page 197) and start combining from that place. Or you can double-stack for two doses, like Power Honey (page 161) and Power Butter (page 161). The goal is to give you the ability to experiment with the adaptogens while also giving you high-functioning, travel-friendly vehicles for them. And you can instantly turn your other foods functional, whether you're baking your own recipes or simply making toast with butter and honey. It's as simple as replacing any other sweetener or fat with these guys.

As for the rest of the recipes, they are designed to be made ahead, in big batches, and all around not overwhelming to make. You could easily swap in other adaptogens—which I've made recommendations for in each recipe—or even other adaptogenic blends. If you've got your eye on Horny Goat Weed Brownies (page 184) but want to go all in on beauty instead, just use the beauty blend instead of the epimedium (for sex). You are also invited to play with other ingredients. For example, once you make Amla, Strawberry, Rose Sorbet (page 123), you'll see how you can make one-step sorbet in the blender and can now start to play with other flavor combinations so you're not stuck in the world of strawberries and rose. If you have an overabundance of fruit in your kitchen, or something looks really great at the farmer's market, you can think about using your blender and an adaptogen you're intrigued by to make new treats.

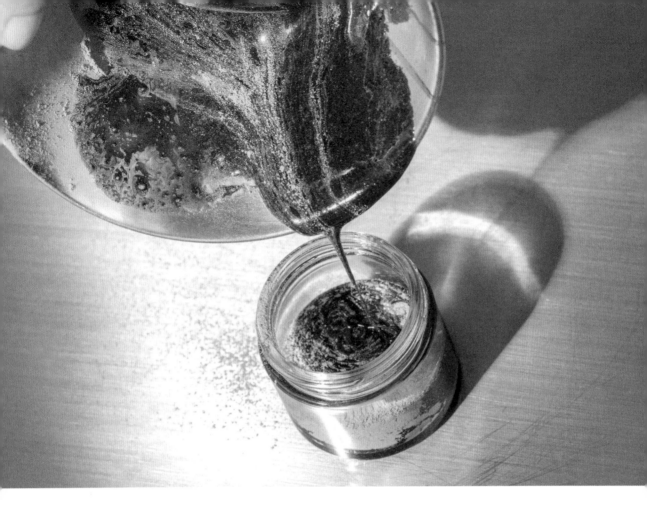

NOTES ON BUTTERS AND HONEYS

If you want to make a recipe zero-glycemic or vegan, just omit the honey, add a few drops of stevia, and use coconut oil.

I chose to use coconut oil or ghee in the recipes because they're the perfect vehicles for blending the adaptogens into drinks, and they can go either sweet or savory; you can use them for cooking or baking. However, any of the butters can be made using the same amount of any other seed, nut, or fat. Simply swap in your butter or fat of choice using the same measurements.

For those heeding Ayurvedic advice, be mindful that honey is considered toxic when heated. Simply add your honey to a tonic that is warm versus hot, or, if you prefer a piping-hot tonic, you can instead use your butter and sweeten with something else.

Keeping Food
Highly Functional

You'll notice that these recipes are all grain-free and lower-glycemic. That's for good reason: In addition to delivering the power of adaptogens, I want these recipes to also nourish your body. Both sugar (naturally occurring and processed) and grains can exacerbate an autoimmune condition, adrenal dysfunction, and hormone-related weight gain because they contribute to inflammation, candida growth, hormone fluctuation, and stress on the organs. I also call for using plenty of healthy fats—nut and seed butter, coconut butter, avocado—to help the body assimilate the adaptogens. These measures are all designed to reduce stress on the body and embrace the pillars of functional medicine.

It used to be that our food was medicine *and* a meal, especially in Ayurvedic and traditional Chinese medicine practices. Now we've found ourselves in a time of excess, and for many of us it's the root of dysfunction. That's not to say that a return to more functional practices means giving up food as pleasure. I was a chef; I have an intense connection to food as an emotional experience, as a pleasurable experience, as a communal experience, and as an art form. I also have these functional eating habits that have delivered me from mental and physical lows. What I've noticed is that these two paths blend. The functional food has become extremely pleasurable, and it's a new kind of pleasure—a deeper pleasure, a more sustaining pleasure. There's absolutely still room in my life for things that are not functional, like pizza and ice cream—and I don't feel bad about that in moderation. But the pleasurable-functional foods in my diet have completely changed my relationship to what I eat, and truly my entire life.

FIVE POWERFUL PRINCIPLES

1

Get Raw to load up on enzymes, minerals, and phytonutrients (anything not heated above 115 degrees).

2

Get Alkalized to balance your pH and tame inflammation (the greener the better).

3

Mineralize to give your brain and body the nutrients they need to thrive (activated nuts and seeds—especially sesame and pumpkin seeds—pink salt, cacao, and leafy greens).

4

Eat Good Fat to nourish your brain, nervous system, and hormones (raw plant fats like avocado, coconut, nuts, seeds, and olive oil).

5

Slow Your Glycemic Roll by limiting sugar in all forms (experiment with monk fruit or stevia and eat ferments to reduce cravings).

Finding Your Rhythm
with These Recipes

In terms of when to enjoy your new roster of healing treats, go back to what your existing habits are. Are you someone who champions the first meal of the day? (I am!) Go for the granola or pancakes. Or add a spoonful of honey to your smoothie. If you're not into breakfast but take a to-go cup of coffee, blend in a spoonful of butter. Then throughout the day, listen to your body for when you need another hit. It's no different from that voice that tells you that you're thirsty, hungry, tired, or need protein. If you give your body enough time using the adaptogens, it will start to crave them, whether it's for a spirit lift, an energy boost, or something to help you wind down for bedtime. These recipes are built to deliver regular help from the adaptogens without having to overhaul your daily practices.

MAKING COMMUNAL HABITS

A great way to get more adaptogens into your life is to tag-team the ritual. In my house, whoever doesn't have to be out the door first makes a double batch of tonic and divides it into thermoses for the taking. The same goes for our nighttime ritual of tea or another pre-bed tonic. There's a particular sweetness to partaking in these practices together, and it's completely practical. If you and your friend, roommate, or partner can hack your habits together, you not only get to bond on a new level, but you only have to remember half the time.

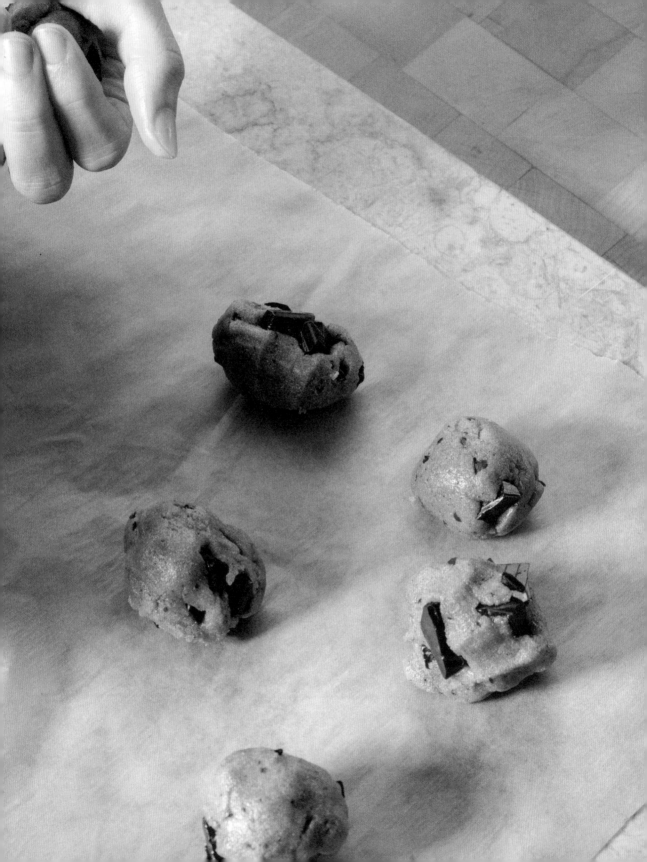

A NOTE ON BIG-BATCH PREPARATION

You'll notice that a number of these recipes can be made ahead of time—in full or in part—stored, and then enjoyed over a long period of time. This is for a couple of reasons. The first is that it means that in one industrious afternoon you really could set yourself up for six months to a year. If you're feeling inspired and find a pocket of time, prepare a handful of these recipes so that these foods are available to you when you need them most—namely, when you don't have any time and when taking care of yourself tends to go out the window. If it's a baked recipe, you can combine the dry ingredients and store them in an airtight container (just make sure to give the jar a good shake before using to redistribute the herbs), then mix in the wet ingredients when ready to cook. You could also bake off a batch of brownies and freeze them until you're ready to enjoy. Chocolates and pops can be stored in the freezer for up to twelve months, and the dough can be made in bulk, kept in the fridge for a month, and rolled at your leisure. And then there are the honeys and butters, which will survive the year if you're not sticking licked spoons or unwashed fingers in them.

Another reason why I'm a fan of piecemeal preparation is because you can more flexibly change the adaptogens to the recipe. If you make a canister of granola or brownie mix without the adaptogens, you can prepare a small batch with your adaptogen of choice at that moment, versus committing to a year of reishi—or you can stack additional adaptogens on top. The same goes for balls—simply make the dough and roll in the adaptogens as enjoyed. Refer to the dosage chart for each adaptogen on page 93.

SPECIAL EQUIPMENT

Silicone Molds for Pops, Gummies, and Chocolates

One of the few pieces of "special" equipment I call for in these recipes is a silicone mold for various gummies, chocolates, and frozen pops. Essentially, it's just to make life easier, since they're easy to use and clean. But please feel free to use a regular ice cube tray for any and all recipes.

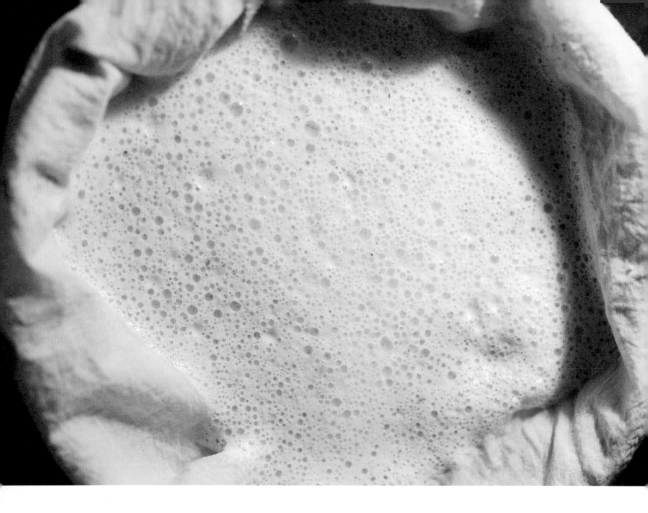

Adapto-Lattes

As you'll see in each chapter, one of my favorite ways to enjoy these adaptogens is to blend them into tonic lattes. There are a number of varieties to play with, but at its simplest, it's warmed milk, slightly sweetened, spiked with adaptogens (or other treasures like collagen, cacao, turmeric, or protein) and blended until rich and foamy. Homemade milks are simple to make (seriously—it's soaking, blending, and straining), are less expensive than store-bought, and offer superior flavor and texture. Make a larger batch at the beginning of the week and you won't miss buying it. Here are a few of my favorite milk staples.

Almond Milk

Almond milk alkalizes and mineralizes the body while providing ample plant protein. If you're feeling industrious, you can save all the pulp, dehydrate it, and use it in any recipe calling for almond flour.

MAKES ABOUT 5 CUPS

1 cup raw almonds

4½ cups water

2 pinches of pink salt

2 teaspoons raw honey (or adaptogen honey) (optional)

1
Place the almonds in a large bowl and add enough water to cover. Soak in the fridge overnight.

2
Drain the almonds and rinse. Transfer them to the bowl of a blender and add the water, salt, and honey, if using. Blend on high for 30 to 45 seconds, until the nuts are broken down and the liquid is milky. Don't over-blend.

3
Strain through a nut milk bag, cheesecloth, or fine-mesh strainer and store in the refrigerator for up to 1 week. Reserve the pulp and dehydrate, if desired.

Hemp and Coconut Milk

Great for metabolism, hormones, and brain function.

MAKES ABOUT 4 CUPS

4 cups water

3 heaping tablespoons hemp seeds

4 teaspoons fresh or frozen young coconut

Pinch of pink salt

1
Combine all of the ingredients in the bowl of a blender.

2
Blend on high for 45 seconds or until smooth. If you have a high-speed blender, you will not need to strain the milk before storing in the fridge. If you don't have a high-speed blender, blend for an additional 45 seconds and strain through a nut milk bag, cheesecloth, or fine-mesh strainer. Store in the fridge for up to 1 week.

Toco Milk

Tocotrienols protect and nourish the skin. When blended into water, they make an effortless milk.

MAKES ABOUT 4 CUPS

4 cups water

½ cup tocos

Pinch of pink salt

1
Combine all of the ingredients in the bowl of a blender and blend for 45 seconds.

2
Store in the refrigerator for up to 1 week.

BEAUTY

BALANCE

Radiant Skin
Healthy Hair
Strong Nails
Clear Eyes
Healthy Gums

IMBALANCE

Lackluster or Troubled Skin
Thinning Hair
Cellulite
Brittle Nails
Puffy Eyes
Inflamed Gums

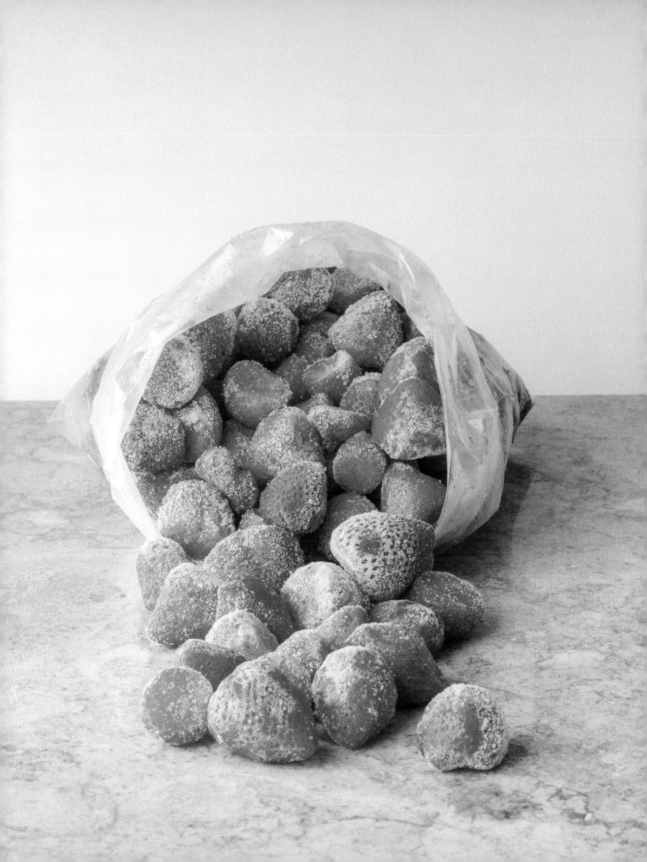

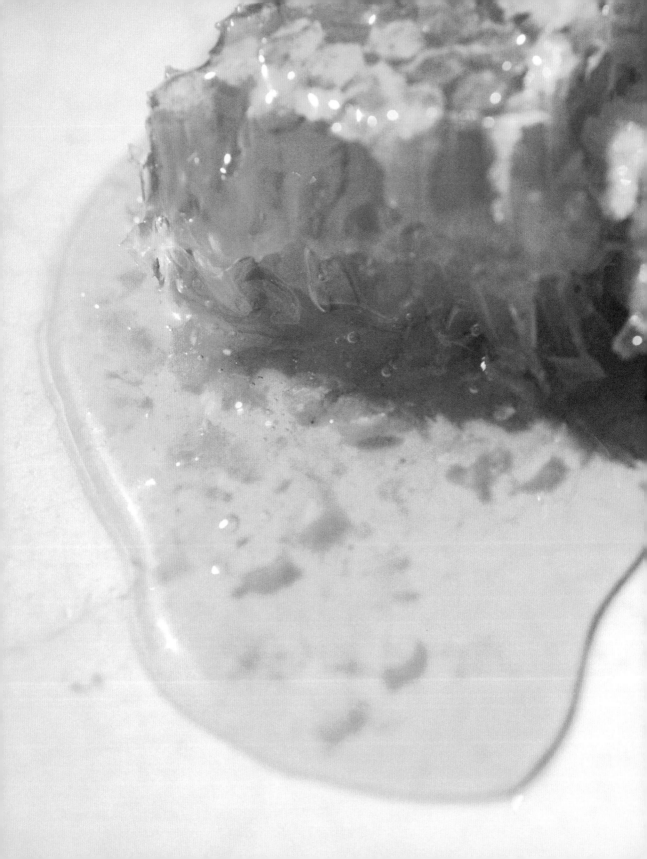

Beauty is a barometer of what is going on inside your body and mind—a mirror of your inner ecology. When we feel our most beautiful on the outside, it's because our bodies are reflecting true harmony within. When your brain and nervous system are organized and calm, your hormones are in balance, your digestive system is optimized, and your spirit is strong, it shows. It's reflected in firm, supple skin with clear, even tone and a glow; thick, healthy hair; strong nails; clear eyes; and no signs of inflammation, dehydration, brittleness, or puffiness. It's the outer manifestation of an inner peace and balance.

That balance is largely threatened by stress, whether it's taxing the lymphatic system—which is at the heart of the body's detoxification protocol—producing sleep-disrupting cortisol, or emotionally separating us from the practices that make us feel good. There are also the effects of "inflammaging," inflammation-induced accelerated aging. In addition to things like environmental pollution, UV rays, stress, illness, and lack of sleep, a major contributor to inflammaging is glycation, or the process where sugar in your bloodstream attaches to proteins and forms molecules that lead to inflammation (breaking down of collagen and elasticity in the skin), hormonal imbalance (weight gain, blemishes, or discoloration), and circulation issues. The adaptogens to call upon—amla, schisandra, tulsi, and shatavari—offer edible radiance. They preserve the body's natural collagen and revitalize hair, skin, and nails. These adaptogenic beauties are rich in antioxidants, and tame inflammation and puffiness.

Amla

Long hailed as a powerful beauty tonic that is rich in antioxidant vitamin C, amla is the great protector of the skin, preserving collagen protein and guarding against the aging effects of free-radical damage. It also actively contributes to beautiful skin by helping to increase elasticity, and its highly astringent and antibacterial properties make it beneficial in combating skin conditions and infections. Amla has also been said to promote the integrity of healthy, strong hair, teeth, and nails.

Minimum daily dosage: ⅛ teaspoon (.50 gram)
Maximum daily dosage: ⅓ teaspoon (1.00 gram)
See also: Power, Spirit

Tulsi

An astringent and a natural antibiotic, this herb is great for anyone suffering from any kind of skin disorder—it kills bacteria on the skin's surface and balances inner-body chemistry to banish acne and soothe irritation.

Minimum daily dosage: ½ teaspoon (1.5 grams)
Maximum daily dosage: 1 teaspoon (3.00 grams)
See also: Brain, Power, Spirit

Schisandra

Once only available to members of the royal courts of China, the schisandra berry has been revered for thousands of years for its ability to make the skin smooth, supple, and radiant. Schisandra builds *wei chi*, or immune defense energy that flows just beneath the skin, while also purifying the liver, which is often the origin of skin issues. It both heals the skin—especially in the case of acne, psoriasis, dermatitis, or other inflammatory conditions—and protects it from damage and radiation exposure. The latter has prompted some to use schisandra as herbal support when undergoing chemotherapy treatment. This berry's overall effect is healthy hair, skin, and nail growth; increased collagen production; plump, hydrated skin; improved skin elasticity; and a glow that emanates from within.

Minimum daily dosage: 1 teaspoon (1.00 gram)
Maximum daily dosage: 2 teaspoons (2.00 grams)
See also: Power, Sex, Spirit

DR. SARA GOTTFRIED

What is beauty?

Beauty is a mirror of your internal ecology, which relates to the way you eat, drink, sleep, move, think, detox, and supplement. In my twenty-five years of functional medicine practice, I've found that beauty evolves from the interdependence of hormones, nutrients, neurotransmitters, microbiome, genetic workarounds, and lifestyle design and redesign.

Genetics certainly plays a role in beauty, but it's small. Only about 10 percent of your risk of disease is genetic; 90 percent is environmental. The same is probably true of beauty. After all, beauty is part of your phenotype or physical traits resulting from the interaction of genetics with the environment, much of which is under your control.

Beauty is created, not bought. That's why self-care and eating foods of various colors are more effective than plastic surgery. That's why exercising every day, modulating stress, eating greens, and dwelling in a state of natural hormonal and homeostatic balance make you more attractive.

Beauty is an expression of soul, not ego. There's no need to improve upon nature. Leave your neurons free to take on weightier matters rather than your jewelry or lipstick. You enhance beauty by being good to your cells.

What are biological factors that disrupt internal and external beauty?

High stress raises cortisol; the internal disruption manifests externally as wrinkles and loss of firmness and elasticity in the skin.

Toxins disrupt key hormones like estrogen, thyroid, and insulin, making you fat, foggy, and rapidly aging.

Food that doesn't suit you due to intolerance or allergy raises cortisol and pokes holes in your gut, over-activating the immune system lying beneath your gut wall.

Poor sleep raises cortisol and makes you hungrier the next day.

Adaptogens
and Weight Loss

When I was in the early stages of figuring out my autoimmune situation, I would occasionally inexplicably gain weight—or at least I thought it was inexplicable until I made the connection between the stress I was experiencing and how my body, specifically my thyroid, was affected. I could actually see the stress in my blood work, and in turn I saw that stress in my body. The key to maintaining a healthy weight isn't just about the foods you eat and the way you move. Managing your stress and your cortisol, on the other hand, is what will lead to hormonal changes that support your healthy weight. What you'll see by feeding yourself these adaptogens is that your stress chemistry will reregulate and in turn your weight will stabilize in a healthy range. If this doesn't move the needle for you, I highly recommend having your blood and hormone panels analyzed by a functional medicine doctor.

The other avenue that stress affects weight is through stress eating. The least effective thing someone could tell you is to just stop snacking. Instead, let's get functional with it. If you know you're stress eating and can't stop, let's replace some of those unhelpful foods with proactive ones that will actually contribute to rebalancing your hormones. Go for your Rhodiola Chocolate Ice Cream (page 144), Tulsi Beauty Jellies (page 124), or Blissy Fig Balls (page 203). Replacing your drug of choice with low-glycemic, functional foods will help you feel more even-keeled and lighter in body and spirit. It's a new take on comfort food.

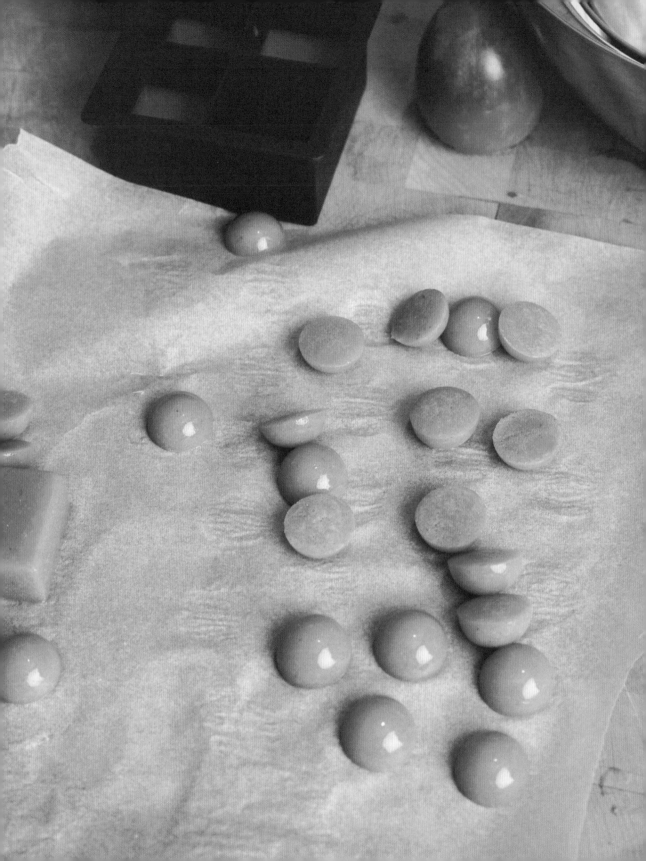

DR. PRATIMA RAICHUR

What is beauty in balance?

One of the most beautiful things about nature is its variation, and that includes us humans and the myriad ways that we may radiate health and beauty. However, there are some universal signs we can recognize as optimal health, even amid all our diversity. With the skin, no matter how thick or thin, no matter how large the pores may be, no matter the shade or tone, and even the age, healthy skin should be clear, shiny, and glowing. Similar traits pertain to healthy hair, shiny and bouncy, and no matter what the texture, and regardless of whether the hair is worn short or long by preference, healthy hair should have the ability to grow. Healthy nails should have the ability to grow and be thick, which is a sign of good calcium and mineral content in the system. Healthy nails should also be pink, which indicates good circulation and hemoglobin. And finally, nails should also have good "half-moons" as a sign of good digestion and healthy thyroid function. Weight is not a measure of health or beauty in its own right, but a range in which a diversity of healthy bodies exists. Instead, we should also be aware of how our systems are functioning, our physical stamina, and our ability to perform daily activities with ease.

What are signs of imbalance?

Stress is a major cause of imbalance and another important reminder of our connection between the mind and the body. While everyone responds differently—depending on their constitution or *dosha*—common signs of imbalance in the skin can include excessive dryness, sagging skin, acne, rosacea, broken capillaries, redness, itching or burning skin, excessive oiliness, clogged pores, and congestion. For the hair and scalp, you may notice imbalances like dryness, dandruff, hair breakage, or trouble growing hair. Watch out for nails with no half-moons, or nails with bumps, lines, or white spots, as well as nails that have difficulty growing. Weight-related imbalances due to stress could result in weight gain from excessive eating, or poor digestion, leading to body aches, joint pain, or poor mobility. Weight loss could also occur due to anxiety, loss of appetite, or discomfort due to heartburn, indigestion, bloating, etc. Emotional stress including fatigue, depression, and lack of motivation can also affect weight. Most important to keep in mind, these symptoms are usually signs of internal imbalances. So if we notice certain imbalances, while there are certainly things one can do externally to mitigate the symptoms, it's important to look deeper within for potential root causes, thought patterns, diet, lifestyle, etc.

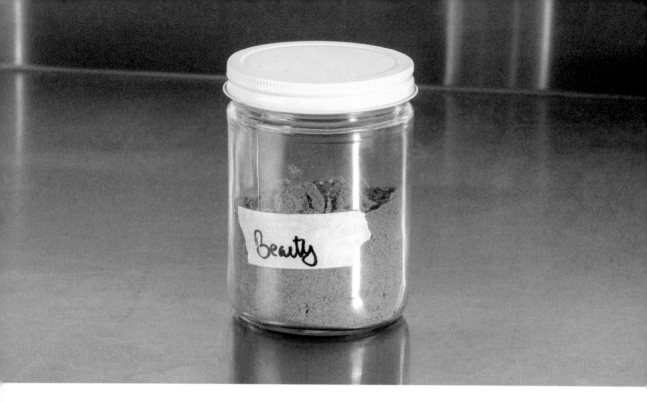

Beauty Mix

Enjoy with water, tea, smoothies, or any other recipe from this book.

DAILY DOSE (2 teaspoons)

⅛ teaspoon amla

1 teaspoon schisandra

¹⁄₁₆ teaspoon tulsi

1
Combine the adaptogens in a small bowl and mix well.

BIG BATCH (30 servings)

3¾ teaspoons amla

½ cup plus 2 tablespoons schisandra

1¾ teaspoons plus ⅛ teaspoon tulsi

1
Mix the adaptogens together and store in an airtight container for up to 1 year.

2
Occasionally mix the batch to make sure the adaptogens are well combined.

Beauty Honey

You may eat this honey straight out of the jar for a whole-body tonifying adaptogenic hit, or wherever else you would like a little sweetness. I like it on yogurt, in iced tea, and mixed into almond butter for a treat.

DAILY DOSE

2 teaspoons Beauty Mix

1 tablespoon raw honey

1
Combine the adaptogens and honey in a small bowl and mix until a thick paste forms.

MONTH SUPPLY

1 Big Batch of Beauty Mix

1½ cups raw honey

1
Combine the adaptogens and honey in a medium bowl and mix with a rubber spatula until you have a thick, even paste. Transfer to a lidded glass jar and store at room temperature. Handled in a sanitary way (i.e., no double-dipping), this will last for up to 1 year.

Beauty Butter

Coconut and its healthy fats and natural antibacterial and antifungal properties make it incredible for skin, hair, and metabolism.

DAILY DOSE

4 teaspoons Beauty Mix

2¼ teaspoons coconut oil or ghee

1
Combine the adaptogens and coconut oil in a small bowl and mix until a smooth paste forms.

MONTH SUPPLY

1 Big Batch Beauty Mix

1½ cups coconut oil or ghee

1
In a double boiler or a heatproof bowl set on top of a simmering pot of water, melt the coconut oil. Remove from the heat and stir in the adaptogens. Let the mixture cool, then transfer to a lidded glass jar for storage. Stir occasionally as the mixture solidifies to ensure even distribution of the adaptogens. Store at room temperature for up to 1 year.

Iced Beauty Matcha

A tonic with a gentle hit of caffeine from matcha, a green tea that is rich with vitamins, minerals, antioxidants, and amino acids. Bump up this recipe by adding a protein powder, tocotrienols (a creamy beauty food derived from brown rice that's like snowflakes of vitamin E), or collagen. Make a quick single serving or make several batches and store them in the fridge for up to 1 week. Enjoy over ice or warm the milk first for a hot latte. For a zero-glycemic version, use 1 tablespoon Beauty Butter (page 119) and stevia.

Makes 1 tonic

1 tablespoon Beauty Honey (page 119)

1½ teaspoons matcha

1 cup milk—I like unsweetened Almond Milk (page 107) or coconut milk

1

Combine all of the ingredients in the bowl of a blender and blend for 30 seconds.

2

Pour over ice and enjoy.

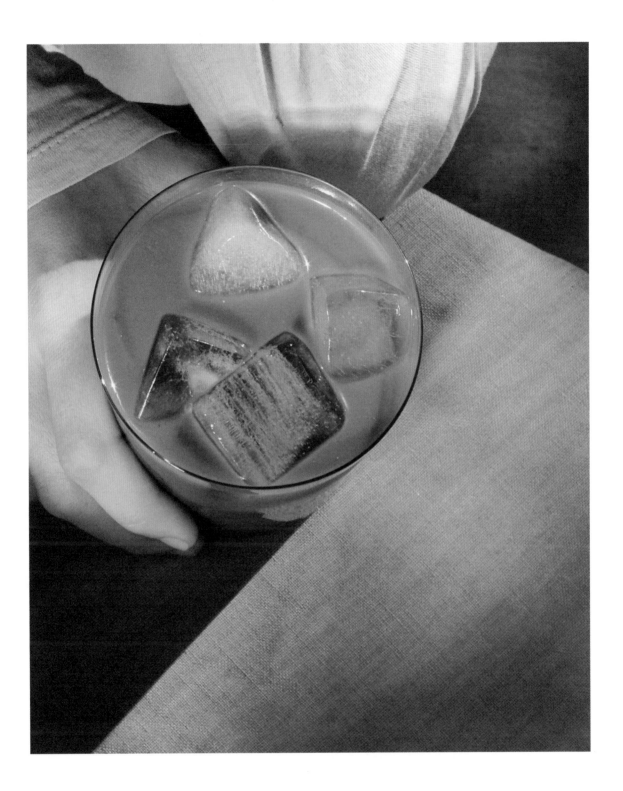

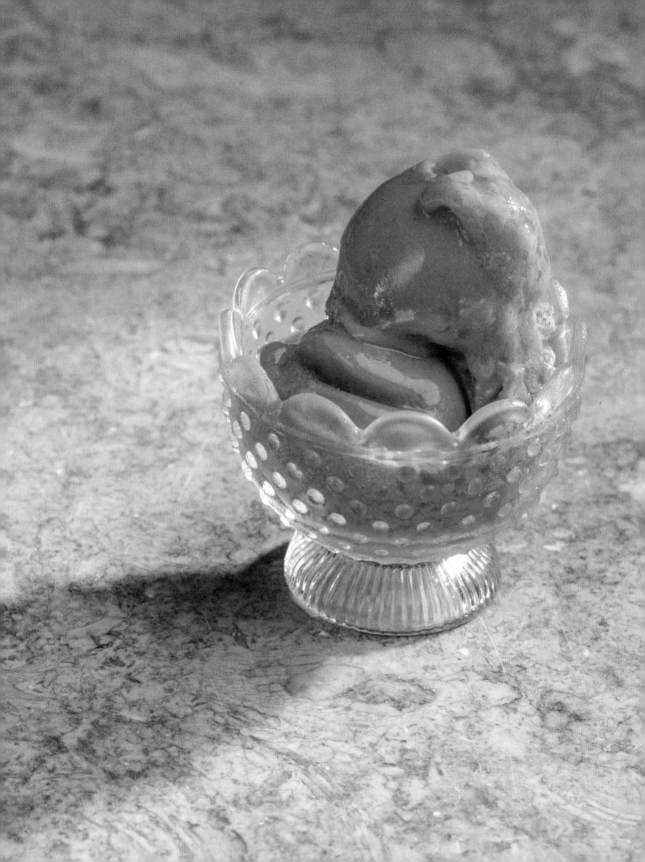

Amla, Strawberry, Rose Sorbet

All you need to make this lusciousness is a blender. It can be made lower-glycemic by using stevia, or you can sweeten it with your adaptogen-infused honey—Beauty Honey (page 119), Power Honey (page 161), Spirit Honey (page 197)—or otherwise. I highly recommend indulging in this fresh while it's whippy and soft, but you could freeze it in an ice cube tray or pop molds for future enjoyment. Other adaptogens that would work well here are schisandra, licorice, shatavari, and cordyceps.

Serves 3

2 cups frozen strawberries

2 tablespoons rose water

1 tablespoon Beauty Honey (page 119) or 3 drops stevia

⅓ teaspoon amla

1

Combine all of the ingredients in the bowl of a blender and blend on high until smooth. If you have a blender with a tamper, you'll want to use it to work the berries down. If you don't, add ¼ cup water to get the puree started. It's best enjoyed straight out of the blender.

2

For big batches, you may store this in the freezer for up to 1 month, but you will need to pull it out and thaw it for 20 minutes to re-scoop.

Tulsi Beauty Jellies

Jellies are a fun and easy way to get a daily dose of adaptogens, and this berry base makes it super versatile for using with other adaptogens—especially amla, schisandra, licorice, ginseng, eleuthero, and astragalus. You can make a single-adaptogen batch, or make a few different kinds of jellies. If using licorice, you'll want to hold off on the sweetener; if using amla, be a bit more generous. Feel free to use gelatin in place of agar-agar if it's what you prefer. And while I call for using silicone candy molds with 2-ounce cups, a small baking dish lined with parchment paper will also work. Just slice the jellies into ½-inch squares once they've set.

Makes eighteen 2-ounce jellies

1 cup raspberries, fresh or frozen and defrosted

1 cup strawberries, fresh or frozen and defrosted

3 tablespoons agar-agar or gelatin

3 drops of stevia or 2 teaspoons honey

1 teaspoon tulsi

1

Combine the raspberries and strawberries in the bowl of a blender. Blend on high for about 30 seconds, until completely pureed. This will lend about 2 cups of berry puree.

2

Strain the puree through a sieve, using a rubber spatula to coax it through. Discard the seeds and set aside 1 cup of the puree. If you have a bit extra (there is variation among the berries of the world), store the remaining puree in the fridge. Use it in smoothies, or freeze for a future batch of jellies.

3

In a small saucepan over low heat, bring 1 cup of water to a boil. Reduce the heat to a simmer, add the agar-agar, and whisk for 5 minutes. Remove the pot from the stove and let the mixture cool, about 10 minutes.

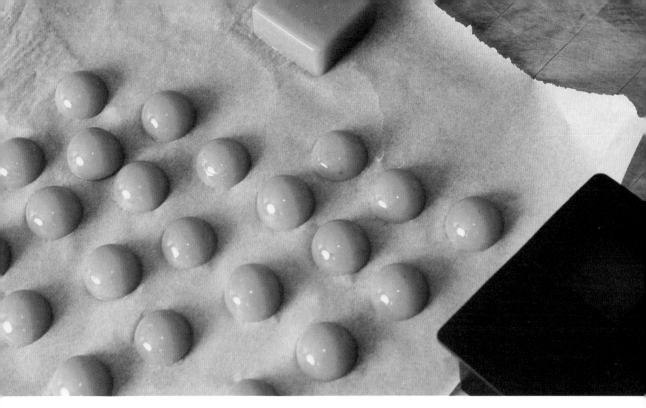

4

Whisk in 1 cup of berry puree, your sweetener of choice, and the tulsi. Whisk vigorously until all of the ingredients are evenly incorporated.

5

Pour the berry base into candy molds, an ice cube tray, or a small baking dish lined with parchment paper. Transfer to the fridge and allow the jellies to set for about 1 hour. Store in the fridge for up to 1 week.

Schisandra Beauty Balls

I call for using sesame butter here because it's high in iron and B vitamins, both important parts of your beauty health, though you could substitute Beauty Butter (page 119). For an extra boost, roll these in bee pollen. This sesame–dried apple–cherry base would also work well with tulsi, amla, licorice, mucuna, and cordyceps.

Makes 10 to 12 balls

1 cup dried apple rings

1 cup unsweetened
dried cherries

½ cup raw sesame butter

1 tablespoon schisandra

½ cup hemp hearts

1

Combine the apple rings and cherries in the bowl of a food processor and pulse until a fruit "dough" is formed. Transfer to a large mixing bowl.

2

Add the sesame butter and schisandra to the dough mixture. Using a wooden spoon, massage the ingredients together until completely and evenly combined. Place the hemp hearts in a small bowl and set aside.

3

Roll the dough into 10 to 12 truffle-size balls. Roll each ball in the hemp hearts until completely covered, then gently press with your hands to "set" them in.

4

Store the balls in the fridge in an airtight container for up to 1 month.

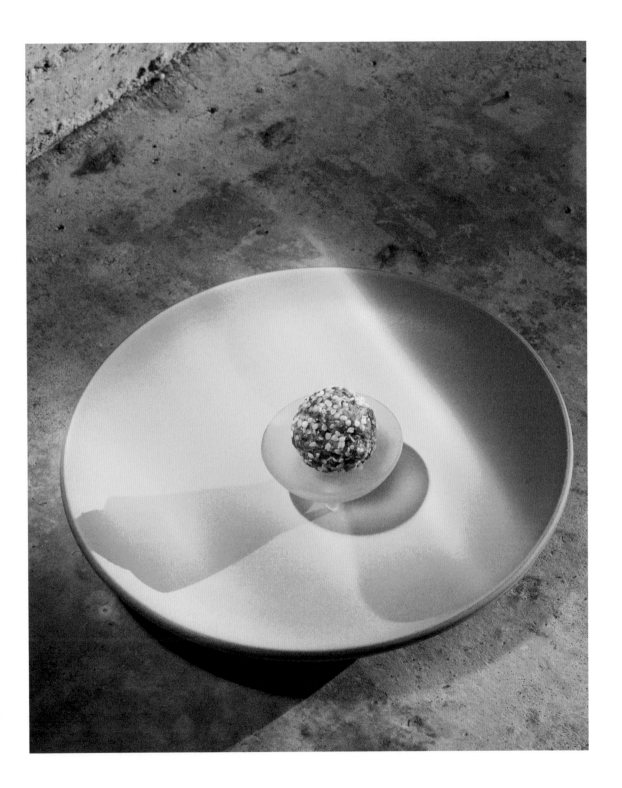

Beauty

BRAIN

BALANCE

Fluidity and Nimbleness
Capacity to Learn and Retain New Information
Manageable Range of Emotions
Velocity, Sharpness, Quickness of Decisions
Clarity of Thought
Good Memory Recall and Retention
Adaptability to Change

IMBALANCE

Mental Fog
Lack of Attention; Easily Distracted
Overstimulation
Rigidity of Thoughts
Feelings of Overwhelm
Sluggishness
Forgetfulness

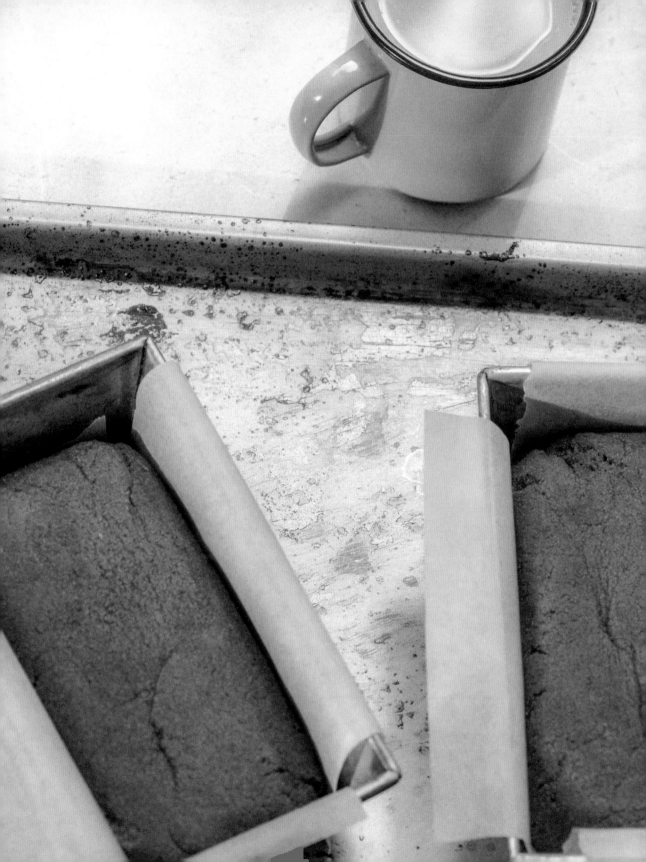

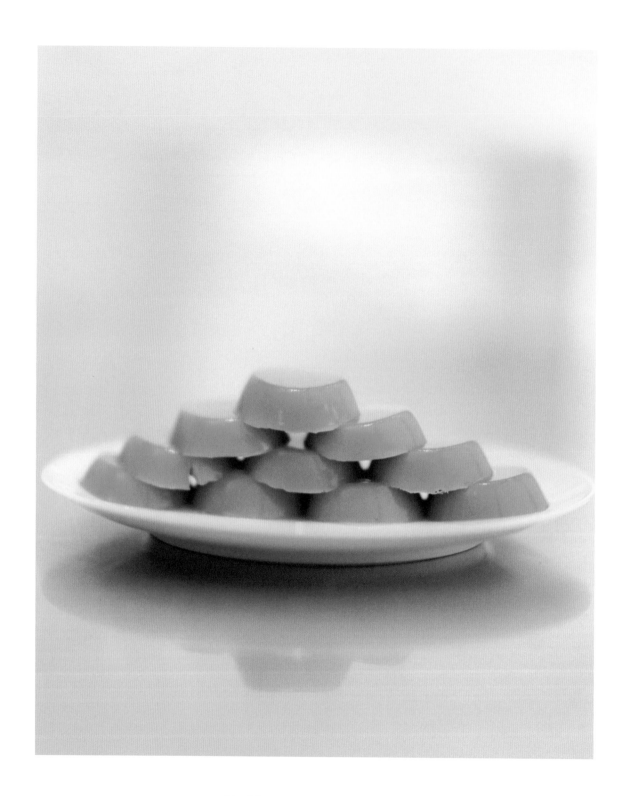

The ability to multitask is an absolute necessity, but it takes its toll on the body. When your brain is overstimulated with clutter and noise, it's difficult to make concise decisions, and mental exhaustion and fatigue follow suit. Stress hormones like cortisol and adrenaline only obfuscate matters further, leading to a brain fog that settles over every aspect of your life. Because your brain is the messenger, and the conductor, if you have compromised brain function, the rest of the body suffers, whether it's flagging energy, erratic emotions, disrupted sleep, or no libido. An overworked, undernourished brain can't detox the way it needs to, it can't properly catalog incoming information, and it's certainly not up for expansive thought. But when the brain is healthy, your entire being comes into focus. A supple brain bathed in plenty of oxygenated blood is a key to longevity, sending good, strong messages to all of your other physiological players.

The herbs in this chapter are highly active nootropics, edible cognitive superchargers that help your brain keep up. They enhance circulation to improve attention and memory; keep the mind clear, centered, and focused; reduce mental fatigue and fog; and protect the nervous system from damage. Because the brain drives the human machine, these herbs support the entire body. Expect strengthened immunity, invigorated energy stores, deeper sleep cycles, and aroused fire.

Ginseng

By stimulating brain cells, ginseng helps with cognitive perception and concentration, leading to improved focus and the ability to problem solve. Though this root can be energizing mentally, it has a calming effect on the body. It's been used to treat insomnia by offering deep, restorative sleep, as well as to improve mood and reduce anxiety by balancing the adrenals. Ginseng has also been shown to be effective as a natural treatment for ADHD and hyperactivity.

Minimum daily dosage: ¼ teaspoon (1.00 gram)
Maximum daily dosage: ¾ teaspoon (3.00 grams)
See also: Power, Sex

Reishi

Reishi supports membrane detoxification and mitochondrial health, in turn leading to increased energy production and focused cognitive function. Reishi helps the nerves transmit information, improving basic brain function. Its anti-inflammatory properties help cultivate more intense concentration and sharpen memory, while its cardiovascular-pumping encouragement supplies the brain with the fresh blood and oxygen it needs to function at peak ability.

Minimum daily dosage: 1 teaspoon (1.00 gram)
Maximum daily dosage: 4 teaspoons (4.00 grams)
See also: Power, Spirit, Dream

Rhodiola

Not only does rhodiola lower stress-triggered cortisol, it's also rich in natural dopamine and serotonin. These neurotransmitters help improve overall brain function, sharpen focus, and enhance memory while also balancing the emotions and tickling happiness and pleasure centers. When taken regularly, this herb radiates positivity throughout the mind and body.

Minimum daily dosage: 1/16 teaspoon (.15 gram)
Maximum daily dosage: 1/8 teaspoon (.34 gram)
See also: Power, Spirit

What is a healthy brain?

The brain is the most important organ in the body, yet the most neglected. I've learned the most about the biology of impeccable brain function by studying the structure and function of *disorder*. The main disorder that I've found in my patients is daily stress, which creates profound erosion in the mind, the spirit, and the body—and when even one of those areas declines, it impacts the other two. In most of my patients, the balance tips in favor of excess wear and tear rather than growth and repair.

When I think about a healthy, glistening, wise brain, it's a brain in equilibrium, a state of stable balance with equal input from diverse physiologic factors, from mundane to mystical. The brain in homeostasis is not angry, reactive, toxic on alcohol or fluoride or lead, inflamed, depressed, overwhelmed, anxious, or hijacked by stress. To me, the biology of the brain rests upon three key principles: homeostasis, growth, and repair. That is true from cell to soul.

In my thirties and coping with new motherhood, my brain was a hot mess. I was making more wear-and-tear hormones compared to growth-and-repair hormones. I was in the red with my thoughts and behaviors. The root cause? I was skimping on sleep, traveling too much, stressed out, drinking too much wine at night, and, as a consequence, my blood sugar was high (not diabetes but prediabetes). I was moody, was worried too much about situations that didn't belong to me, and had obsessive thoughts about my weight, brain fog, and spotty memory. I couldn't maintain focus and organization like I could when I was younger. I felt overwhelmed.

At the time, my biology showed up on tests as a failure state: my cortisol was too high, my other sex hormones were too low, and my thyroid was slow. The control state in my brain couldn't keep up with the stress inputs, so the outputs suffered. I suffered, along with my husband and family.

Out of necessity, I sought ongoing functional medicine protocols aimed at addressing the root cause of my health issues, and, finally, clear boundaries on the nonnegotiables: love, connection, sleep, service. I also found relief in nature and mysticism. I ultimately recognized that homeostasis isn't staying-the-sameness, it's a process of adapting in a beneficial, intelligent way to the twists and turns of life while keeping my biological foundation rock solid.

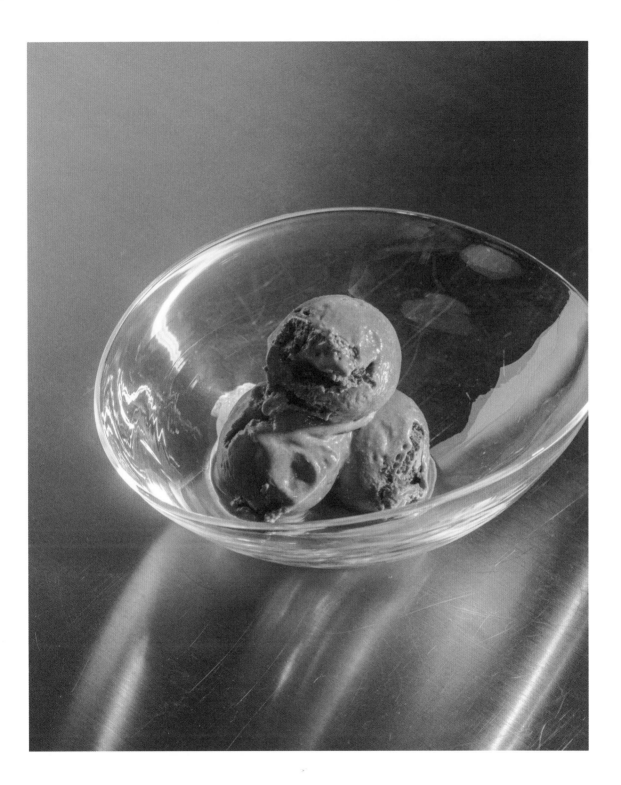

Brain

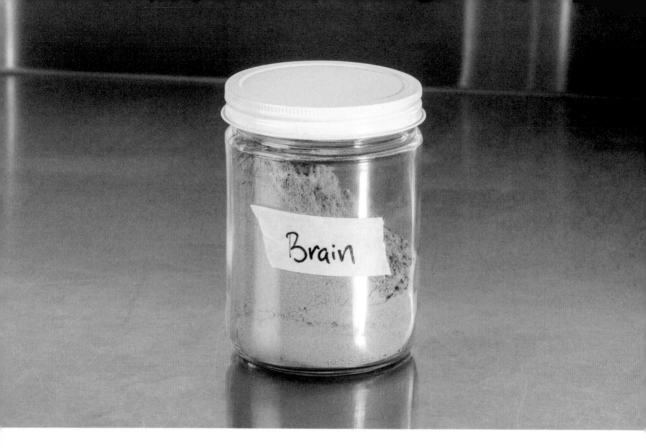

Brain Mix

DAILY DOSE (1¼ teaspoons)

¼ teaspoon ginseng

¹⁄₁₆ teaspoon rhodiola

1 teaspoon reishi

1
Combine the adaptogens in a small bowl and mix well.

BIG BATCH (30 servings)

2 ½ tablespoons ginseng

1 tablespoon rhodiola

10 tablespoons reishi

1
Mix the adaptogens together and store in an airtight container for up to 1 year. Enjoy with water, tea, smoothies, or any other adaptogen-friendly recipe from this book.

2
Occasionally mix the batch to make sure the adaptogens are well combined.

Brain Honey

Eat this honey straight out of the jar or use it wherever you'd like sweetness and an adaptogenic, nootropic hit. I like it in hot chocolate, coffee, on apples, and with walnut butter for extra braininess.

DAILY DOSE

1¼ teaspoons Brain Mix

1 tablespoon raw honey

1
Combine the adaptogens and honey in a small bowl and mix until a thick paste forms.

MONTH SUPPLY

1 Big Batch Brain Mix

1½ cups raw honey

1
Combine the adaptogens and honey in a medium bowl and mix with a rubber spatula until you have a thick, even paste.

2
Transfer to a lidded glass jar and store at room temperature. Handled in a sanitary way (i.e., no double-dipping), this will last for up to 1 year.

Brain Butter

This is a bitter butter that I like to use in my hot tonic drinks by blending it with water instead of adding milk. The recipe calls for coconut oil, which is rich in medium-chain triglycerides (MCTs), otherwise known as brain fuel.

DAILY DOSE

1¼ teaspoons Brain Mix

2¼ teaspoons coconut oil or ghee

1
Combine the adaptogens and coconut oil in a small bowl and mix until a smooth paste forms.

MONTH SUPPLY

1½ cups coconut oil or ghee

1 Big Batch Brain Mix

1
In a double boiler or a heatproof bowl set on top of a simmering pot of water, melt the coconut oil or ghee. Remove from the heat and stir in the adaptogens. Let the mixture cool, then transfer to a lidded glass jar for storage. Stir occasionally as the mixture solidifies to ensure even distribution of the adaptogens. Store at room temperature for up to 1 year.[11]

Brainy Coffee

Caffeine can actually be good for the brain—it's a beneficial psychoactive that enhances how neurons communicate with one another. This in turn can improve various aspects of brain function such as memory, mood, reaction times, and general cognitive abilities. This is a particularly great tonic for those who include butter coffee as part of their intermittent fasting, or those who religiously drink coffee in the morning with no ill effect. If, however, you are experiencing acute stress, exhaustion, adrenal fatigue, or an autoimmune flare-up, then caffeine should be the first thing to go. In that case, substitute cacao in place of the coffee.

Makes 1 tonic

One 8-ounce cup coffee—I use a French press and make a pretty weak coffee, as I find it only beneficial if used in moderation, like an herb itself

1 tablespoon Brain Butter (page 137)

3 drops stevia or coconut sugar to taste

1

Blend all of the ingredients on high and get busy!

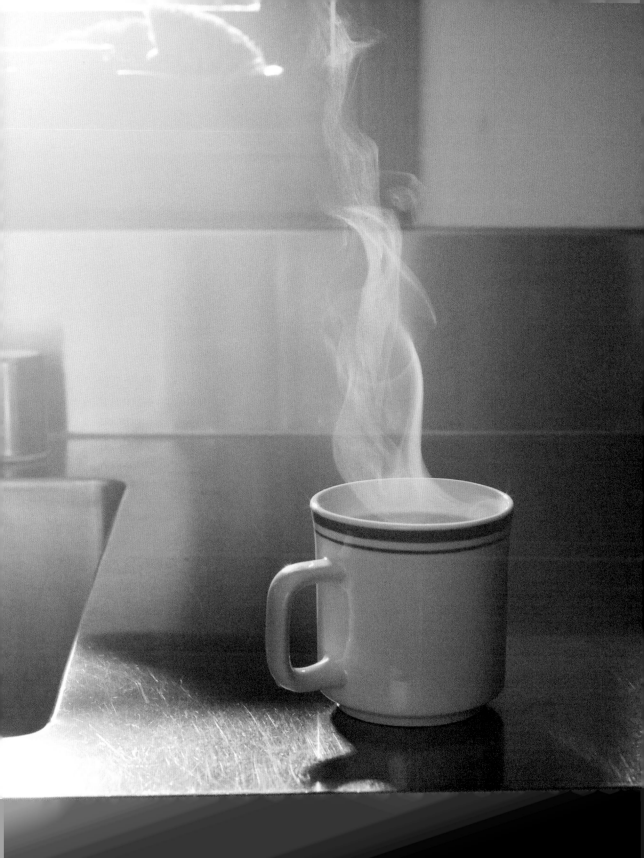

Savory Reishi Broth

This can be a new kitchen staple, perfect in a mug—used as a base for a veggie or noodle soup, or as a cooking liquid for veggies, quinoa, or beans.

Serves 6

10 yellow onions, peeled and quartered

1 head garlic, cloves smashed with a knife and peeled

One 2-inch fat and juicy piece of ginger, peeled with a spoon and sliced into eighths

1 tablespoon coconut oil

6 quarts water

10 dried shitake mushrooms

1 strip of kombu

2 tablespoons reishi

Pink salt to taste

1

In a large stockpot over medium-low heat, sweat the onions, garlic, and ginger with the coconut oil. Stir often for about 8 minutes, making sure not to brown or burn anything.

2

Then add the water, mushrooms, and kombu. Bring to a boil, reduce heat to low, and simmer for 3 hours. Strain the broth and return it to the stockpot on the stove. Add the reishi and salt. Stir until the salt is dissolved. Serve in a mug or in a bowl, store for later, or use as a base for a heartier soup to come. Store the soup for up to 5 days in the refrigerator or for many months in the freezer.

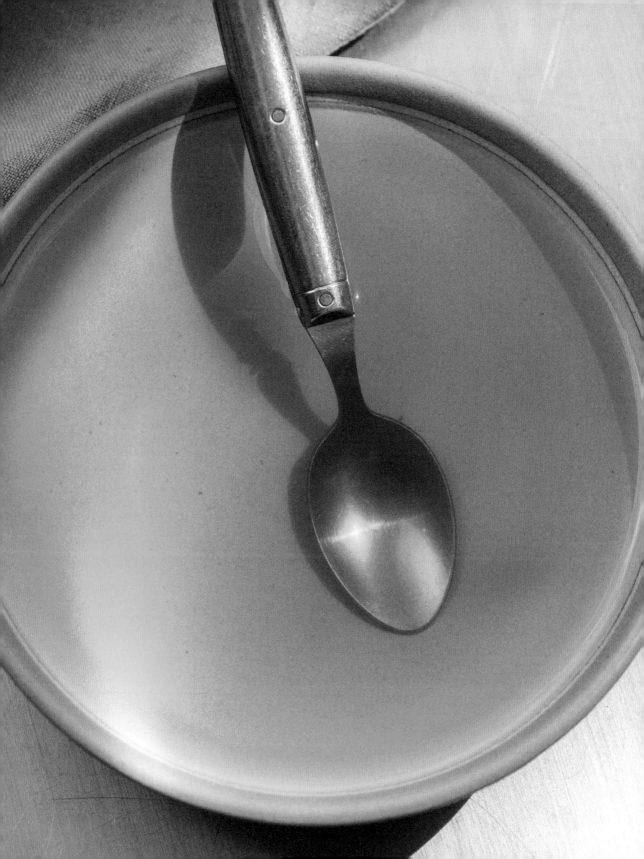

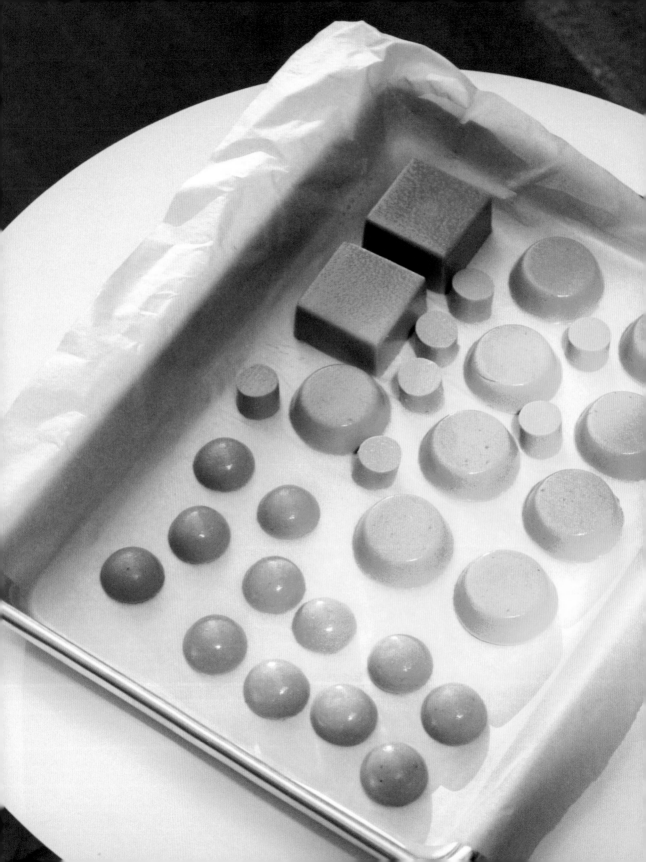

Cold-Brew Ginseng Jellies

For when you need a morning or midday bump. Other adaptogens that would work well here are reishi, mucuna, and shatavari. Feel free to use gelatin in place of agar-agar if it's your preference.

Note that this recipe calls for coconut milk—I prefer fresh, but if we're getting real about these recipes, a canned version is also perfect.

Makes 20 jellies

1¼ cups cold-brew coffee

¼ cup agar-agar

¼ cup coconut sugar or 6 drops stevia

1 cup coconut milk

1½ tablespoons ginseng

1

In a small saucepan, bring the cold brew to a simmer over low heat. Stir in the agar-agar and sugar and whisk for 5 minutes as the mixture simmers.

2

Using a rubber spatula, transfer the coffee mixture to the bowl of a blender, making sure to get every last drop. Add the coconut milk and ginseng and blend on low speed just until the mixture is combined. You don't want to aggressively blend or you'll end up with bubbly jellies.

3

Tap the bottom of the blender on the counter to release any trapped air and pour the mixture into candy molds, an ice cube tray, or a small sheet pan lined with parchment paper.

4

Transfer to the fridge to set, at least 1 hour. If making these in a sheet pan, slice into twenty ½-inch jellies once set. Store in the fridge for up to 1 week.

Rhodiola Chocolate Ice Cream

Cacao is an incredible brain food that optimizes chemistry and gives you an extra hit of mental energy and clarity. Combined with avocado and coconut milk—both great brain fats—this is a particularly great treat for when you want to keep the mental fire burning. It's also low-glycemic (or zero-glycemic if using stevia instead of Brain Honey [page 137]), which means no sugar-induced brain fog. Enjoy scooped directly into a bowl, or freeze it in pop molds or in an ice cube tray. You can enjoy the cubes in a smoothie with almond milk and protein, toss them into iced coffee, or blend them into cold brew with a splash of almond milk for a frozen coffee drink. Other adaptogens that pair well here are mucuna, reishi, shatavari, cordyceps, eleuthero, and astragalus.

Serves 4

One 13.5-ounce can full-fat coconut milk

1 medium avocado, pitted and scooped out of skin

½ cup cacao powder

¼ cup coconut nectar or maple syrup, or for a zero-glycemic version, use stevia to taste, about 5 drops

½ teaspoon raw vanilla bean powder or vanilla extract if you can't find raw powder

¼ teaspoon rhodiola

1

Combine all of the ingredients in the bowl of a blender with ½ cup water. Blend on high for 20 seconds.

2

Transfer to an ice cream maker and churn per the manufacturer's instructions. Or pour into pop molds or an ice cube tray. Freeze until solid.

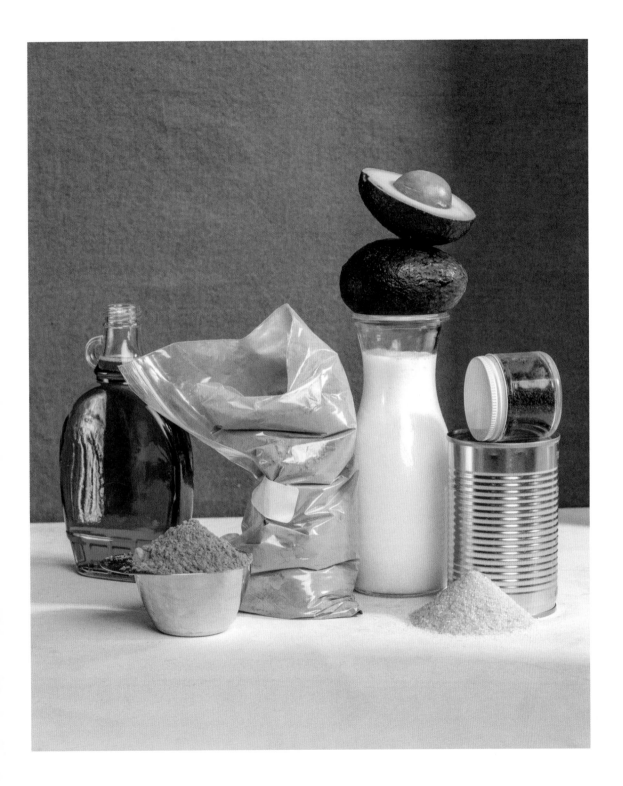

Brain

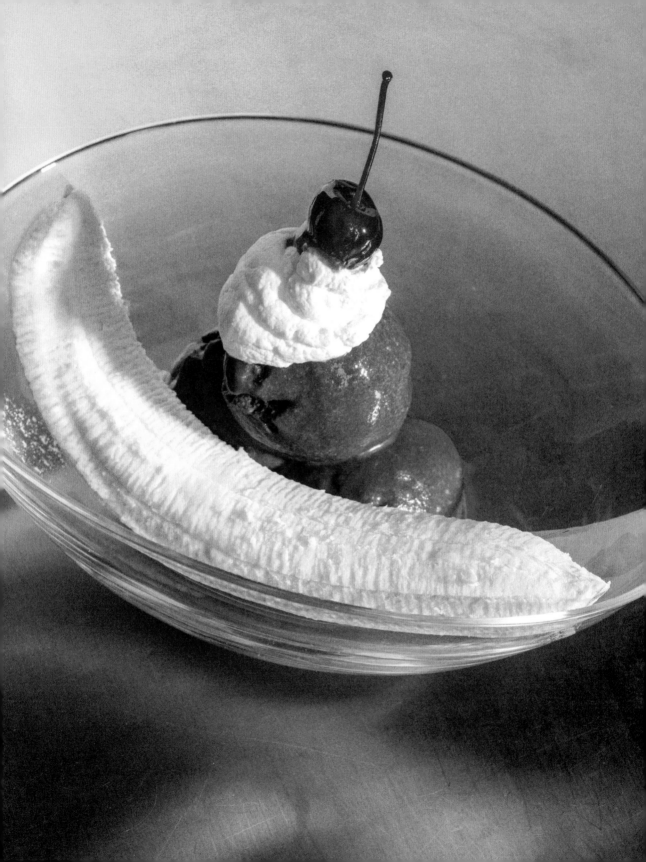

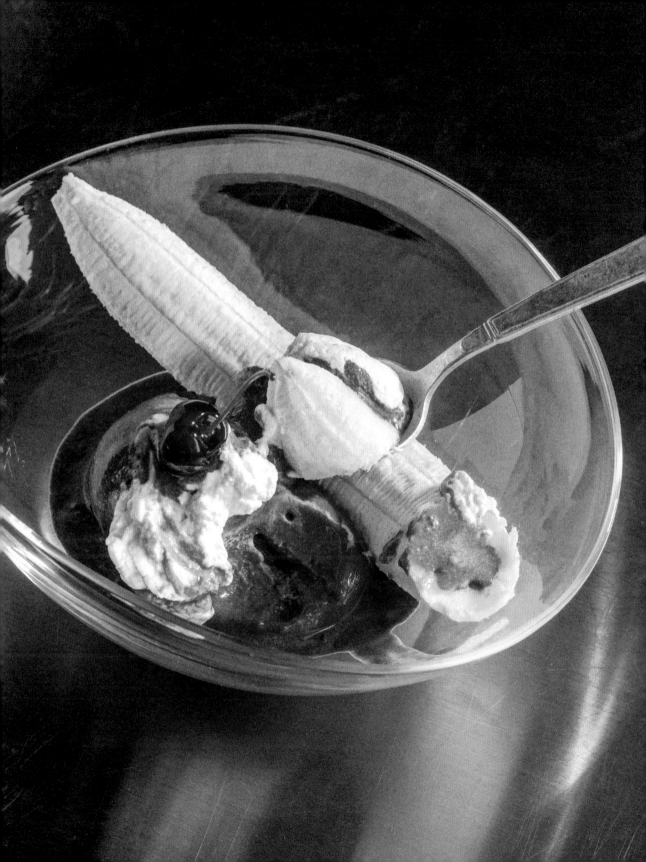

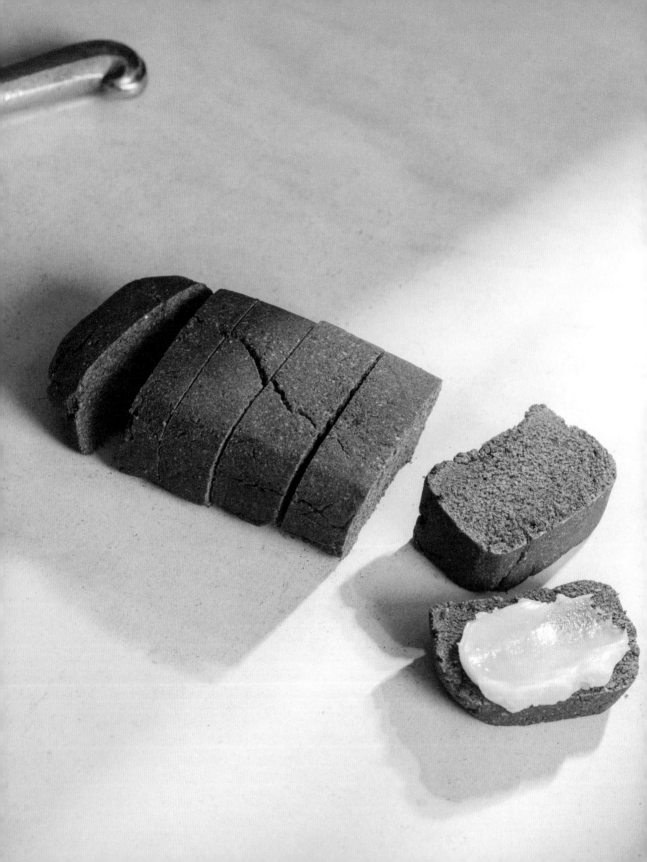

Queen Healer Bread

Give me Queen for breakfast, lunch, and dinner, toasted and topped with ghee, please. It's dense, not too sweet, and stays moist on the counter for days. I really love this one; please make her! Ashwagandha, cordyceps, epimedium, and mucuna would also work well here.

Serves 8

1½ cups almond flour

1 cup cassava flour

¼ cup cacao powder

3 tablespoons reishi

1 teaspoon baking powder

1 tablespoon raw vanilla bean powder or vanilla extract if you can't find raw powder

Pinch of pink salt

½ cup maple syrup

2 tablespoons ground flaxseeds or 2 large eggs

1

Preheat the oven to 350°F. Line a 9 × 5-inch loaf pan with parchment paper and set aside.

2

Combine the almond flour, cassava flour, cacao, reishi, baking powder, vanilla, and salt in the bowl of a food processor and pulse until combined. Add the maple syrup and either the flaxseeds plus 6 tablespoons of water or the eggs. Pulse until a dough forms. Transfer the dough to the prepared loaf pan. Bake for 25 minutes, until firmed up.

3

Allow the bread to cool, and either slice warm or rewarm in the toaster to order. Anoint with butters and/or honeys of choice.

POWER

BALANCE

Deep-Rooted Confidence

Courage

Living on Offense Instead of Defense—and Conquering Your Daily Life

Strong Resilience Against Allergies and Illness

IMBALANCE

Feeling Defeated

Low Energy

Long Recovery Time for Sickness, Wounds, or Workout

Allergy Flare-Ups

Burnout

Adrenal Fatigue

Weak Immunity; Catching Every Flu that Comes Around

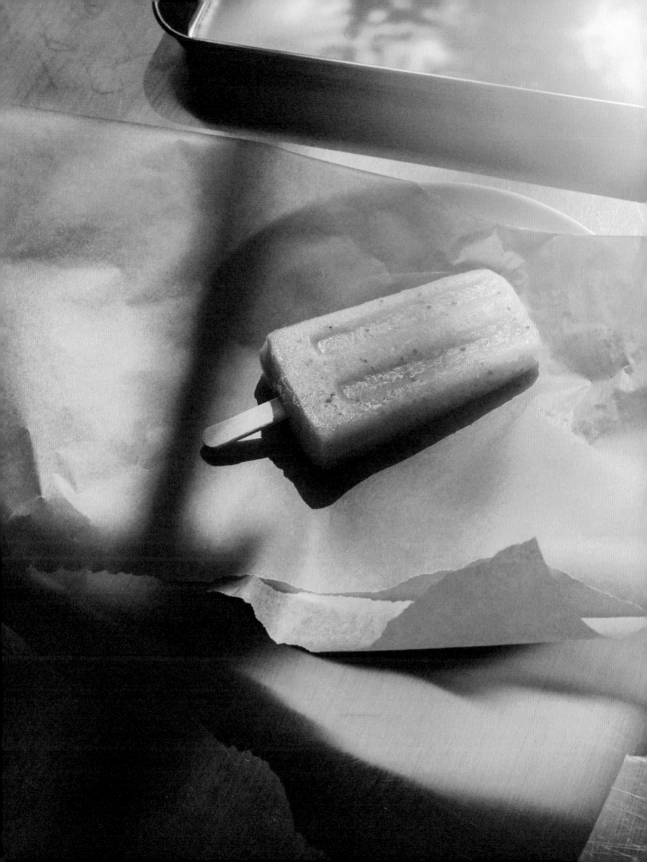

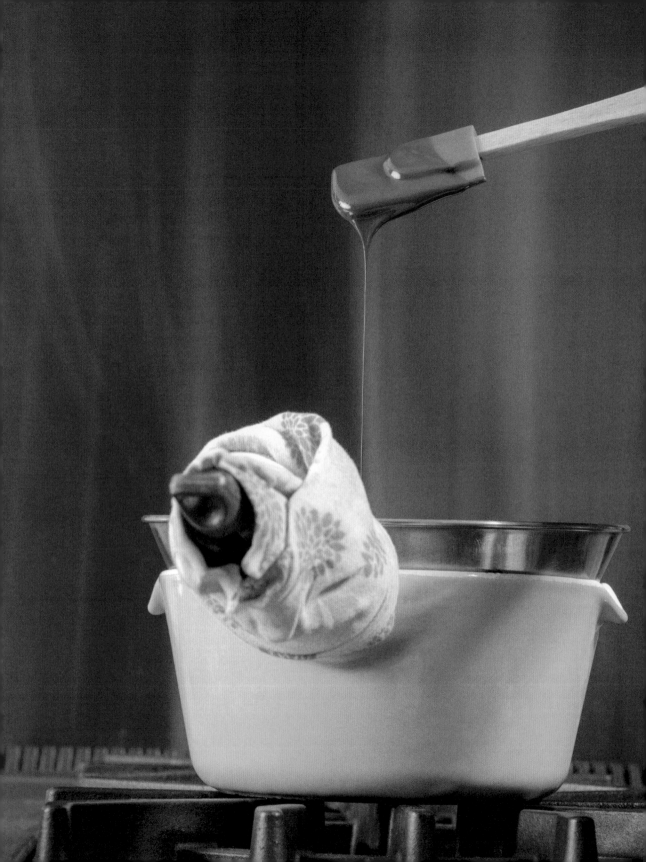

I equate power—endurance, stamina, and strength—with immune function and relaxedness, because they are all intimately intertwined. When you nourish your life-force and replenish your adaptive energy reserve, you bring yourself into a balanced place of true power and longevity; increased energy; optimized recovery (whether from physical activity, travel, or illness); and protection from things—bacterial, viral, energetic—that hold us back from victory.

The herbs in this chapter are your proactive immunity protocol. Turn to them when allergies flare, immunity is weakened, or there are other signs that your adaptive energy reserves are low and need replenishing. It's edible energy that offers whole-body support and resilience for whatever comes your way.

Astragalus

Astragalus is a potent immune booster and rejuvenator, and has long been celebrated as a longevity herb by Taoists in China. Its high concentration of antioxidant compounds helps it tame inflammation, fend off virus- and bacteria-caused illness (it's great taken if you think you're coming down with a cold or flu), calm the allergic response, and repair free-radical-caused oxidation (stress-related wear and tear on the body). It's also been demonstrated to stimulate telomerase, an enzyme that repairs DNA sequences in our cells, which naturally degrade over time. This makes astragalus an essential part of a longevity regimen. Astragalus has long been used to heal wounds, as well as reboot the body after a serious illness or other forms of stress, including chemotherapy. In traditional Chinese medicine, astragalus is said to protect lung energy, and modern research has confirmed its positive effect on the lungs, easing breathing for those with asthma, allergies, or respiratory infections and clearing congestion in the wake of illness. It's also the great defender of the cardiovascular and nervous systems thanks to its beneficial effect on circulation, sending oxygenating blood and rousing energy body-wide. The result is increased stamina and overall physical power.

Minimum daily dosage: 1 teaspoon (2.25 grams)
Maximum daily dosage: 2 teaspoons (4.50 grams)
See also: Brain, Spirit

Eleuthero

Moderating both glandular and hormonal output while also strengthening cells, eleuthero effectively balances the whole body, especially the nervous and immune systems. Used in Russia for the last century to help improve stamina and endurance in athletes, eleuthero helps maintain energy and ward off fatigue. It's also particularly effective in helping the body to cope with extremes in environment. It's an immunity must when the seasons start to change.

Minimum daily dosage: 1 teaspoon (2.00 grams)
Maximum daily dosage: 2 teaspoons (4.50 grams)
See also: Brain, Spirit

Cordyceps

Cordyceps's longtime reverence as a longevity tonic comes from its remarkable ability to multitask. Believed to be key to immortality, Christian, Hindu, and Chinese people have traditionally used the mushroom in spiritual ceremonies. Cordyceps is nourishing for the whole body, enhancing athletic performance, energizing the systems, and boosting your immune system.[12] Studies suggest that cordyceps's ability to improve physical abilities, endurance, and stamina is because it can help increase the body's ATP stores, an essential source of energy during exercise, helping athletes take on tougher and longer feats.[13]

Cordyceps supports the cardiovascular system and better blood circulation, which in turn contributes to improved stamina and overall physical strength, in addition to smoother recovery after exertion. It can also improve respiratory health and increase lung capacity, making it a great supplement for endurance and vitality.

Cordyceps is also considered a natural "immunopotentiating drug," meaning it enhances and strengthens the immune response. Cordyceps directly stimulates the production of NK cells, or "natural killer" cells, which are the body's fiercest defense against infection and illness. They help rearm the immune system after a serious illness or infection and can help subdue autoimmune disorders, particularly by controlling the inflammation and tissue damage that naturally happens during the immune response. While studies have more recently examined cordyceps's ability to strengthen immune function—particularly in the cardiovascular, respiratory, endocrine, and reproductive systems—it's been used for centuries to improve respiratory and heart health, replenish oxygen uptake, detoxify the body, prevent certain types of cancer, slow the aging process, and keep the body energized and insulated from the effects of stress.

Minimum daily dosage: 1 teaspoon (1.00 gram)
Maximum daily dosage: 1 tablespoon (3.00 grams)
See also: Brain, Sex

DR. FRANK LIPMAN

What is physical power?

Power—including recovery and healthy stress management— is what I refer to as "resilience" and is determined by daily practices that restore and support us rather than wear us out. This may include regular exercise, a daily meditation practice, spending ample time in nature, prioritizing sleep, eating the right foods, and/or connecting with loved ones or a higher power.

Travel and Power

Travel, even for pleasure, can be a form of stress. It combines the physical tax of airplanes with things like jet lag, germ exposure, dietary complications, and sleep disruption. Travel is best enjoyed with the support of Power herbs eleuthero, cordyceps, and astragalus, in addition to rhodiola and licorice. You'll find recipes here using these herbs that are particularly easy to take with you and make delicious travel companions.

Exercise and Power

Power adaptogens and exercise are a dynamic duo because these plants boost stamina and endurance while aiding recovery time. They are particularly helpful if you don't have an innate interest in exercise or a regular movement practice and need help with momentum. Moving the body is excellent for circulation; detoxification; oxygenation; and feeding the brain, spirit, and muscles. But as good as exercise can be for you, it can also be overwhelming. Working out too frequently and too aggressively for your body can be a recipe for elevated cortisol that may wreak hormonal havoc. There was a time when I thought I had to work out three to five times a week no matter what in order to manage stress and stay healthy. What I found was that high-intensity exercise combined with a demanding work schedule, parenting, and not sleeping enough was a huge contributor to systemic inflammation, exhaustion, and depletion. I was denying the part of myself that was saying, "Hey, I'm tired! I'm inflamed!" I couldn't pull back from the rigid regimen. What I've found is that hormonal balance plays the biggest role in my physical body. If your hormones aren't balanced, you'll see your metabolism slow and puffiness creep in.

This is definitely not to say that you shouldn't exercise—moving your body is incredibly beneficial to all systems. I'm suggesting that you find a form of movement that serves you best. People often forget how incredible walking is. And I don't know anyone who has been negatively affected by stretching and deep breathing. You don't need to be sweating profusely and freaking your adrenals out in order to reap the benefits of exercise. If you do feel invigorated and strong by a tougher workout, then this message is not meant for you. Just don't forget to listen to your body. If you're feeling puffy, exhausted, or anxious, then maybe a high-intensity program isn't giving you what you need at the moment. Give your body some time and space to rest (and let the adaptogens support and rebalance you). When you're feeling better, slowly incorporate the elements of working out that you enjoy most.

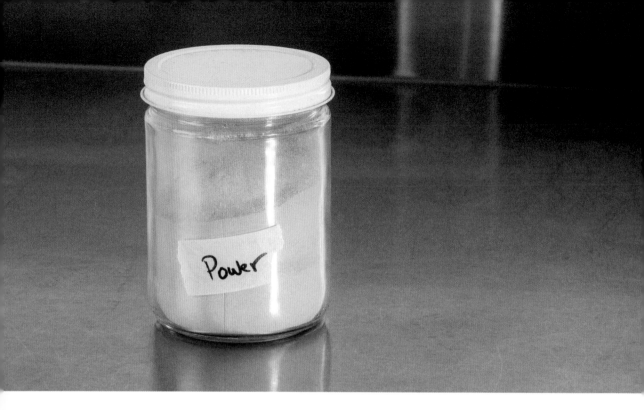

Power Mix

DAILY DOSE (1 tablespoon)

1 teaspoon astragalus

1 teaspoon cordyceps

1 teaspoon eleuthero

1
Combine the adaptogens in a small bowl and mix well.

BIG BATCH (30 servings)

½ cup plus 2 tablespoons astragalus

½ cup plus 2 tablespoons cordyceps

½ cup plus 2 tablespoons eleuthero

1
Mix the adaptogens together and store in an airtight container for up to 1 year. Enjoy with water, tea, smoothies, or any other adaptogen-friendly recipe from this book.

2
Occasionally mix the batch to make sure the adaptogens are well combined.

Power Honey

I love a spoonful of this honey before outdoor activities, and I'll make a couple of doses rolled in hemp seeds for an adventure. It's perfect in iced tea with lemon or mixed into chocolate. Use wherever you would like a little sweetness, energy, recovery, or an immunity boost.

DAILY DOSE

1 tablespoon Power Mix

1 tablespoon raw honey

1
Combine the adaptogens and honey in a small bowl and mix until a thick paste forms.

MONTH SUPPLY

1 Big Batch Power Mix

1½ cups raw honey

1
Combine the adaptogens and honey in a medium bowl and mix with a rubber spatula until you have a thick, even paste. Transfer to a lidded glass jar and store at room temperature. Handled in a sanitary way (i.e., no double-dipping), this will last for up to 1 year.

Power Butter

I love this butter blended into hot tonics and coffee, and I use it in baking, especially pancakes, granolas, and breads.

DAILY DOSE

1 tablespoon Power Mix

1 tablespoon ghee or coconut oil

1
Combine the adaptogens and ghee in a small bowl and mix until a smooth paste forms.

MONTH SUPPLY

1½ cups ghee or coconut oil

1 Big Batch Power Mix

1
In a double boiler or a heatproof bowl set on top of a simmering pot of water, melt the ghee. Remove from the heat and stir in the adaptogens. Let the mixture cool, then transfer to a lidded glass jar for storage. Stir occasionally as the mixture solidifies to ensure even distribution of the adaptogens. Store at room temperature for up to 1 year.

Milk Chocolate Momentum

Chocolate milk, in one form or another, has been daily pleasure/food/self-help for most of my life. It's definitely evolved, and this is now my favorite way to get the daily dose. Feel free to add protein or maca for extra stamina.

Makes 1 tonic

1 cup milk—I like Almond Milk (page 107)

1 heaping tablespoon Power Honey (page 161)

1 tablespoon cacao

3 ice cubes

1

Combine all of the ingredients in the bowl of a blender.

2

Blend on high for 20 seconds.

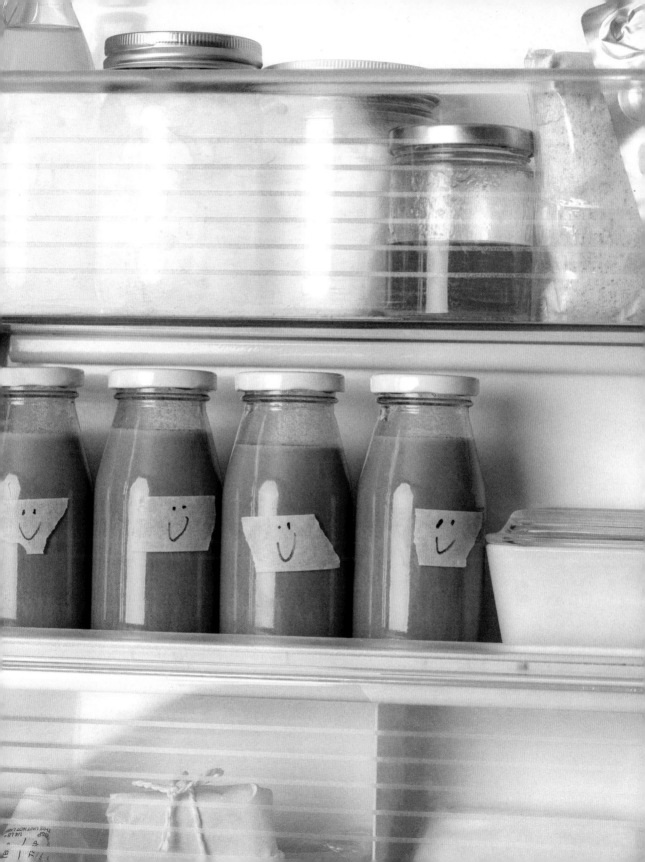

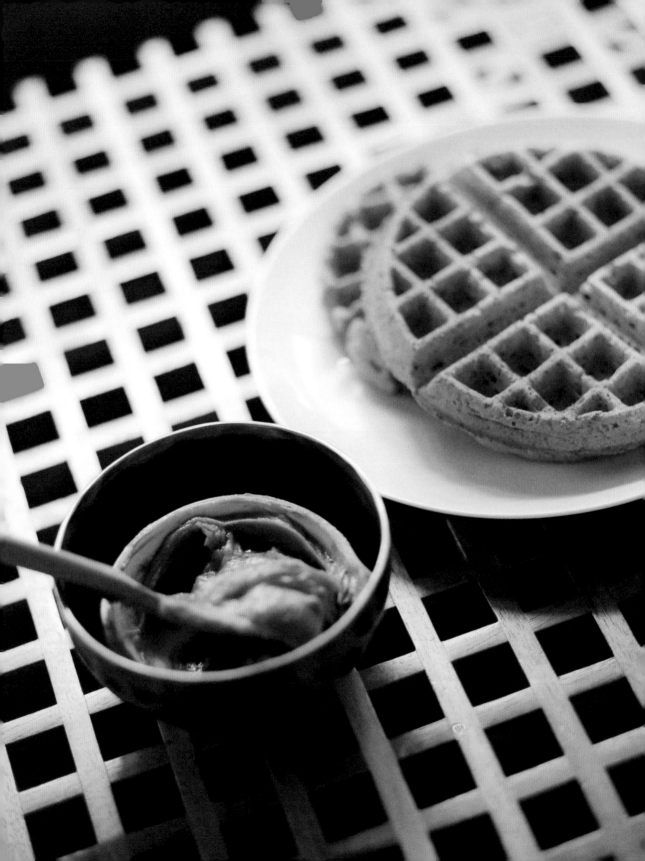

Supershroom Pancakes and Waffles

Success with this lies in making a big batch of the dry mix ahead of time. The dry mix, if stored properly, will last as long as a year (just make sure to mix it thoroughly between each use so the adaptogens are evenly distributed). All that stands between you and a functional feast is adding water and eggs or egg replacement. You may also just spike your grocery store–bought pancake mix or cook off a batch of the pancakes or waffles (cooling and wrapping each individually), so they're ready to be sent out into the day, toasted the next morning, packed into lunches, or frozen for later. Top them with the honey or butter of your choice and call it a meal. Other great adaptogens for this recipe include mucuna, reishi, shatavari, cordyceps, eleuthero, and astragalus.

Makes 4 pancakes

½ cup almond flour

¼ cup cassava flour

¼ cup coconut flour

½ teaspoon raw vanilla powder (optional)

4 teaspoons astragalus

½ teaspoon baking soda

¼ teaspoon pink salt

3 flax eggs or eggs*

½ cup almond milk

Ghee or coconut oil, for cooking

* To substitute eggs: Replace 1 egg with 1 tablespoon ground chia or flaxseeds combined with 3 tablespoons water whisked into a smooth, viscous slurry. Or simply use ½ ripe smashed banana (about ¼ cup).

1

In a medium bowl, whisk together the almond flour, cassava flour, coconut flour, vanilla powder (if using), astragalus, baking soda, and salt.

2

In another medium bowl, whisk together the flax eggs and almond milk. Add the wet ingredients into the dry and whisk until fully combined.

3

Heat a large pan over medium-high heat. (I use a nonstick, nontoxic ceramic one.) Add a liberal amount of ghee or coconut oil, about 2 teaspoons to 1 tablespoon.

4

Spoon batter into the skillet, keeping your pancakes about 3 inches in diameter. They'll be easier to flip. Cook on one side until the edges are golden and the pancakes seem firm enough to flip. Cook for an additional few minutes on the second side.

Spiced Pineapple Pops

These are great to have on hand for when you feel something coming on or are recovering and don't have much of an appetite, blended into a smoothie for an extra boost, used as cubes in iced tea, or enjoyed in the sun—they taste like a party. You could also use schisandra, tulsi, or ginseng.

Makes 6 pops

6 cups pineapple chunks (about 1½ medium pineapples; no need to core the pineapple first)

Juice of 1 lime

1 tablespoon astragalus

¼ teaspoon red chili powder (omit if you don't want a little heat)

1

Combine all of the ingredients in the bowl of a blender and blend for 30 to 45 seconds, until completely smooth.

2

Pour the mixture into Popsicle molds or an ice cube tray and freeze until set, about 3 hours.

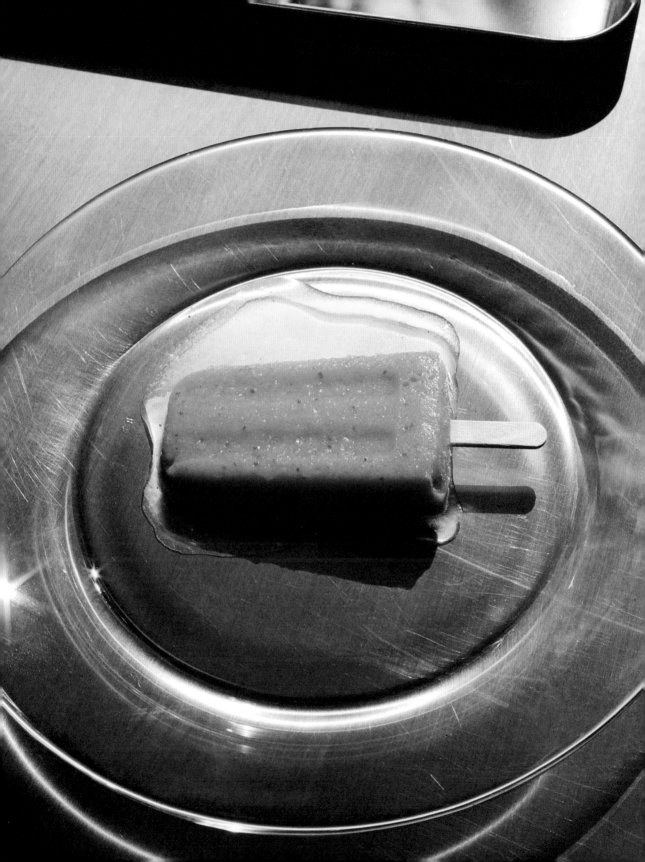

Eleuthero Chocolate Chunk Cookies

This is my favorite cookie ever, grain free, extreme chocolatiness, and deeply nourishing. I like the raw dough as much as the golden baked cookie! Notes: For the chocolate, I like 80% to 100% dark chocolate or hardened and chopped Shilajit Sex Drizzle (page 188).

Makes 8 cookies

1 cup cassava flour

1 cup almond flour

1 tablespoon ground flaxseeds

3 tablespoons eleuthero

½ teaspoon raw vanilla bean powder or vanilla extract

¼ teaspoon baking soda

¼ teaspoon pink salt

¼ cup coconut oil, melted

¼ cup maple syrup

1 cup chopped dark chocolate (two 90-gram chocolate bars; I like 80% to 100%)

1 teaspoon flaky sea salt, for garnish

1

Preheat the oven to 350°F. Line a baking sheet with parchment paper and set aside.

2

In the bowl of a food processor, combine the cassava flour, almond flour, flaxseeds, eleuthero, vanilla, baking soda, and salt with 3 tablespoons water and pulse until well combined.

3

In a medium bowl, whisk together the coconut oil and maple syrup. Add the wet ingredients to the food processor and pulse until the mixture forms a dough. Use a spatula to fold in the chocolate.

4

Form the dough into roughly tablespoon-size balls and arrange them on the prepared baking sheet. For a crispier cookie, gently press the dough to flatten, or leave as is for a chewier consistency.

5

Bake for 35 minutes, until the cookies are firm and golden. Sprinkle with flaky salt. Let the cookies cool completely (ideally on a wire rack) before transferring them to a tightly sealed container. They can be stored at room temperature for up to 5 days.

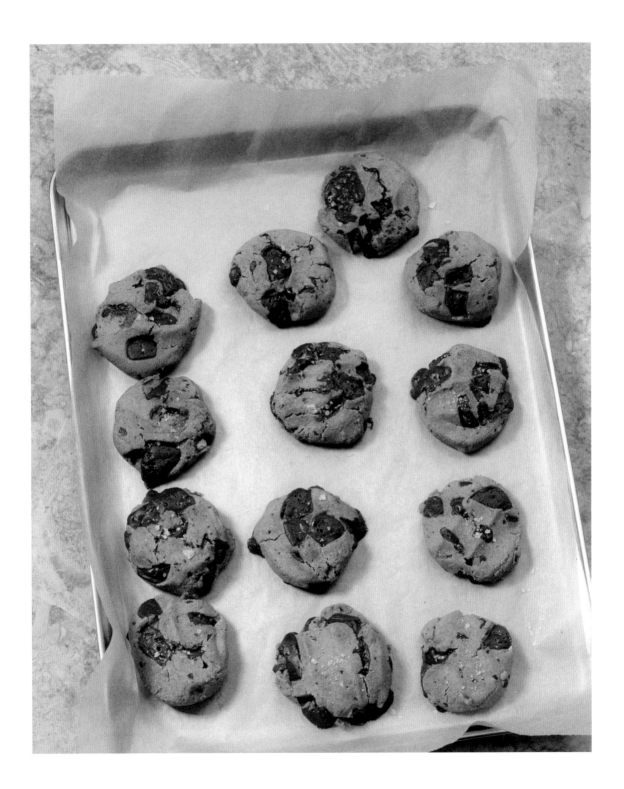

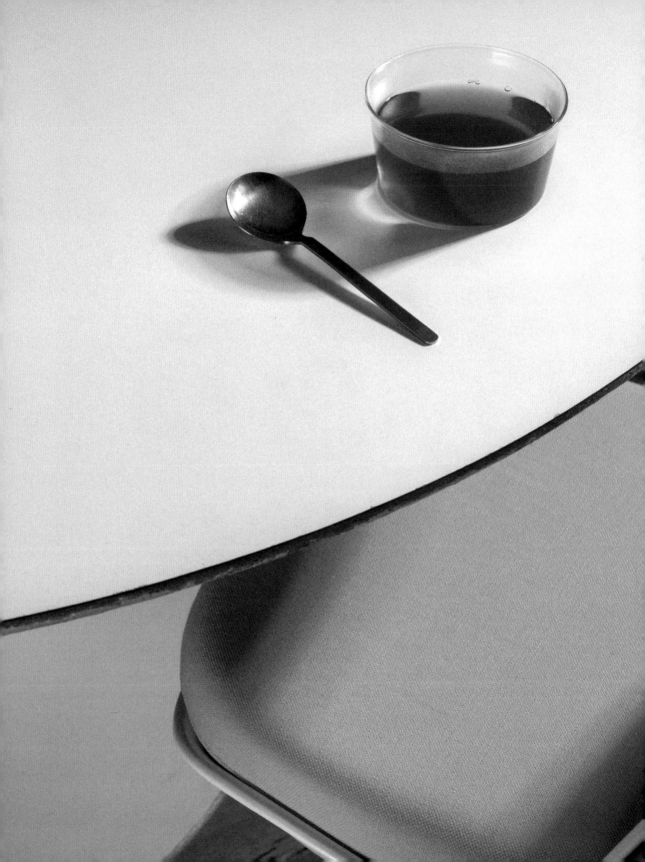

Ginseng Mineral Broth

This is the adaptogenic version of my favorite old-school mineral broth that I would make in my early days of juice cleansing. It's warming, fortifying, mineralizing, and has an extra immunity boost with the ginseng.

Makes sixteen 2-cup servings

6 carrots, washed, unpeeled, and quartered

2 yellow onions, peeled and quartered

1 entire leek, greens included, washed and quartered

4 red potatoes, washed, unpeeled, and halved

2 yams, washed, unpeeled, and quartered

1 bunch celery, washed, leaves included, and quartered

1 head garlic, each clove smashed with a knife and peeled

1 bunch of parsley, washed

2 strips of kombu

15 peppercorns

2 bay leaves

8 quarts water

2 teaspoons powdered ginseng

Pink salt to taste

1

In a large stockpot over medium-high heat, combine the carrots, onions, leeks, potatoes, yams, celery, garlic, parsley, kombu, peppercorns, bay leaves, and water. Bring to a boil, reduce the heat to low, and then simmer for 3 hours.

2

Strain the broth, discard the solids, and return the broth to the stockpot on the stove. Add the ginseng and salt. Stir until the ginseng and salt are dissolved. Serve in a mug or bowl, store for later, or use as a base for a heartier soup to come. Store the soup for 5 days in the fridge or for several months in the freezer.

SEX

BALANCE

Healthy Sexual Appetite
Juices Flowing in Body and Spirit
Effervescent but Stable Energy Level
Fertility and Virility

IMBALANCE

Low Libido, Low Mojo, Lots of Blah
Feeling Uninspired or Unfulfilled
Irregular Menstrual Cycle
Hormonal Acne
Infertility
Signs of Rapid Aging

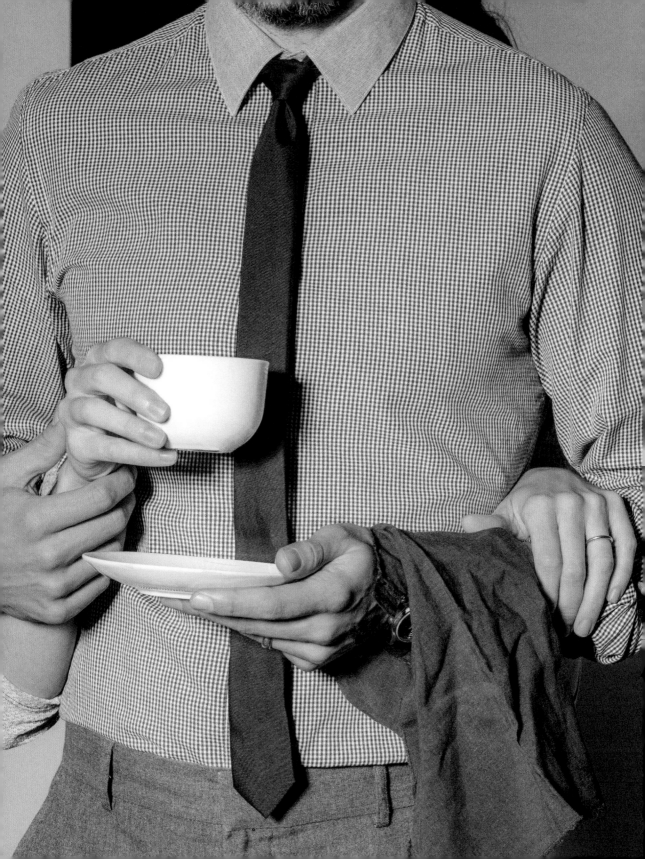

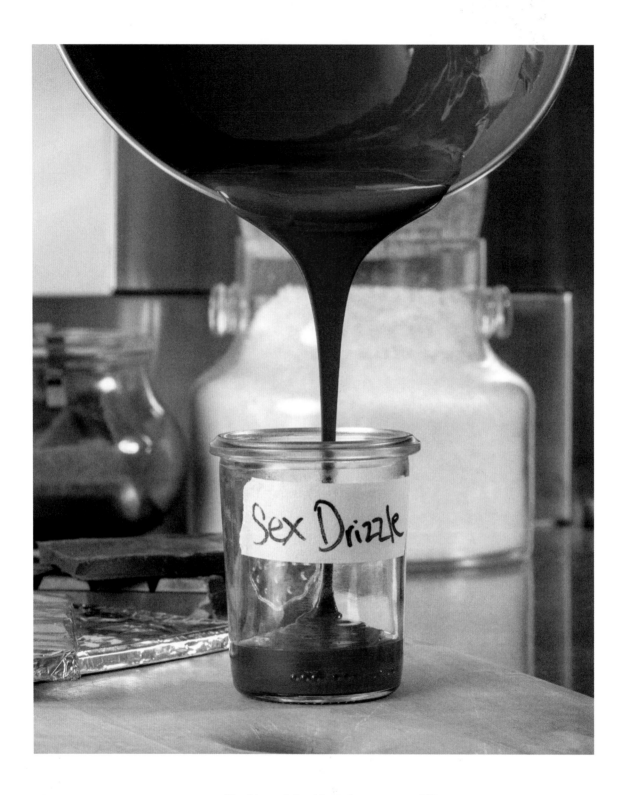

Stress is not seductive—it disrupts sex hormones and dries up juicier inclinations. If we fall under the wave of everyday pressures, we not only hamper our ability to connect with one another, we compromise the flow that contributes to healthy fertility, virility, creativity, and feelings of fulfillment. Our sex hormones affect everything from our drive and thoughts to our appearance. If ravaged by stress, these hormones can no longer keep us vital. We literally dry up, whether it's no longer connecting with things that inspire us or no longer connecting physical arousal with emotional desires.

Healthy sexual energy is creative potential in the body. When you harmonize sex hormones, you feed your life force. You see it manifested in supple skin, thicker hair, and strong teeth and nails—nature's way of signaling vitality. Our blood pumps with vigor, stoking our internal flame, and in our fertile years, our body gets the message that it is safe to receive and nurture a baby. The overall effect is feeling awakened, potent, and on fire.

I highly recommend playing with these adaptogens with a partner—there're something big that happens when two people commit to sexy plants together: The vigor of one is met with the openness of the other.

ALISA VITTI

What does healthy sex look like?

It's libido, mojo, vitality, and creative energy. Biologically, it's about being able to produce appropriate levels of estrogen and testosterone, nitric oxide and oxytocin. Physically, healthy libido is both the interest in engaging sexually—whether solo or with a partner—and the ability to achieve orgasm and climax, which ebbs and flows with your menstrual cycle patterns. Energetically, it's about your capacity to get out of your head and into your body to receive and breathe into the sensations of pleasure.

What does imbalance caused by stress look like?

When cortisol is out of balance, your interest and response sexually can diminish dramatically. It's not all in your head. It will take you longer for tumescence and lubrication to happen, which must precede orgasm and climax. In addition, with elevated levels of cortisol, you'll make less estrogen and testosterone, which further compounds the issue.

What does healthy fertility look like?

This often overlooked key indicator of our overall health as women has finally been acknowledged by the American College of Obstetricians and Gynecologists and is now considered your fifth vital sign after blood pressure, body temperature, pulse rate, and respiration rate. So it's extremely critical for you to be aware of your cycle every month. A healthy cycle is regular and somewhere between twenty-eight and thirty days. Healthy menstruation is red like cranberry juice; it is not clotty, dark, sluggish, brown, spotty, or light, or shorter than three days in duration. Ovulation is regular and marked by obvious, beautiful cervical fluid mid cycle. There are no symptoms of PMS whatsoever.

What does imbalance caused by stress look like?

Cortisol levels rob the body of progesterone, as progesterone is molecularly similar to cortisol and can be substituted when the adrenals are struggling to keep up with the demand. Without enough progesterone to balance estrogen, you can have any and all PMS symptoms, from acne, to bloating, to mood swings, to cramps, and more. You can also have longer cycles and brown staining at the start and end of your bleed. It will also make it more difficult for you to maintain a pregnancy.

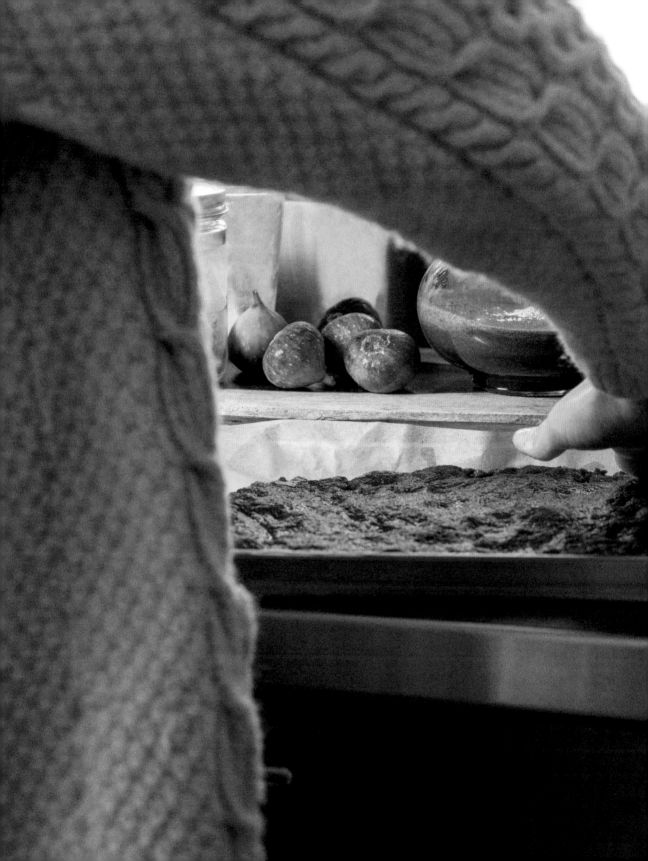

Epimedium

Epimedium, a.k.a. horny goat weed, is among the most potent and prized natural aphrodisiacs: It preps the body for sensual adventures by relaxing muscles, increasing blood flow to the necessary zones, and delivering a powerful dose of icariin nitric oxide, a beneficial compound that stimulates circulation—especially in the sexy regions. Said to address erectile issues in men, epimedium has been shown to have similar effects to prescription drugs like Viagra.[14] For women, it helps send all the right nectars to the clitoris and vagina for engorged pleasure. But epimedium isn't all playtime—rich with phytoestrogens, epimedium is a powerful hormone regulator that helps soothe PMS and menopause and discourage diseases caused by hormonal imbalance, like osteoporosis.

Minimum daily dosage: 1/16 teaspoon (.20 gram)
Maximum daily dosage: 1/3 teaspoon (1.00 gram)
See also: Brain, Power

Shilajit

Long used as an aphrodisiac, shilajit is a champion of fertility and libido. It balances systems throughout the body and boosts testosterone, cultivating an increased sexual charge in men and women. it has also been used to support both ovum and sperm health.

Minimum daily dosage: 1/16 teaspoon (.22 gram)
Maximum daily dosage: 1/4 teaspoon (1.00 gram)
See also: Brain, Power

Shatavari

Shatavari has been used for thousands of years in Ayurveda and translates to "having one thousand husbands." Studies have concluded that the herb is rich in the compounds shatavarin and sarsasapogenin, which are considered precursors to female sex hormones. Shatavari has the power to balance hormones and literally becomes the lifeblood of the reproductive system. This incredible herb is a boon to women in all stages of life, from the very first cycle to completion in menopause. It helps regulate ovulation, soothe PMS symptoms such as cramps, bloating, and irritability (while also providing a dose of folic acid to help prevent anemia), enhance fertility (Ayurvedic texts claim it gives women the ability to produce thousands of healthy ova), prepare the body for carrying and birthing a child by nourishing the womb and reproductive organs, discourage miscarriage, increase lactation, and aid postpartum healing. It can promote healing of conditions such as endometriosis and PCOS (polycystic ovary syndrome) and support women who suffer from low natural estrogen levels owing to menopause, hysterectomies, or oophorectomies. And then there are the incredible effects of optimized hormones that keep membranes (from face to yoni) supple and lubricated and fires stoked (for men and women).

Minimum daily dosage: ⅛ teaspoon (.40 gram)
Maximum daily dosage: ¼ teaspoon (.80 gram)
See also: Beauty, Power

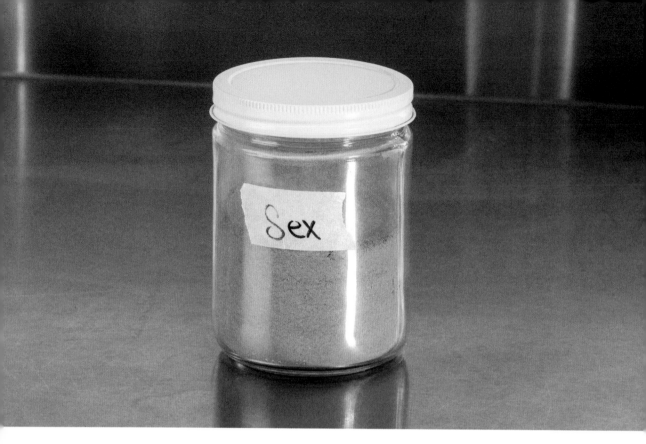

Sex Mix

DAILY DOSE (⅓ teaspoon)

¹⁄₁₆ teaspoon epimedium

⅛ teaspoon shatavari

¹⁄₁₆ teaspoon shilajit

1
Combine the adaptogens in a small bowl and mix well.

BIG BATCH (30 servings)

1¾ teaspoons epimedium

3¾ teaspoons shatavari

1¾ teaspoons shilajit

1
Mix the adaptogens together and store in an airtight container for up to 1 year. Enjoy with water, tea, smoothies, or any other adaptogen-friendly recipe from this book. Occasionally mix the batch to make sure the adaptogens are well combined.

Sex Honey

DAILY DOSE

⅓ teaspoon Sex Mix

1½ teaspoons raw honey

1
Combine the adaptogens and honey in a small bowl and mix until a thick paste forms.

MONTH SUPPLY

1 Big Batch Sex Mix

1 cup raw honey

1
Combine the adaptogens and honey in a medium bowl and mix with a rubber spatula until you have a thick, even paste. Transfer to a lidded glass jar and store at room temperature. Handled in a sanitary way (i.e., no double-dipping), this will last for up to 1 year.

Sex Butter

This is a supreme daily butter that I use for energy and hormone balance, whether it's in my hot tonic drinks or coffee, or mixed with Sex Honey and cacao and slathered on toast as a chocolate spread!

DAILY DOSE

⅓ teaspoon Sex Mix

1½ teaspoons ghee or coconut oil

1
Combine the adaptogens and ghee in a small bowl and mix until a smooth paste forms.

MONTH SUPPLY

1 cup ghee or coconut oil

1 Big Batch Sex Mix

1
In a double boiler or a heatproof bowl set on top of a simmering pot of water, melt the ghee. Remove from the heat and stir in the adaptogens. Let the mixture cool, then transfer to a lidded glass jar for storage.

2
Stir occasionally as the mixture solidifies to ensure even distribution of the adaptogens. Store at room temperature for up to 1 year.

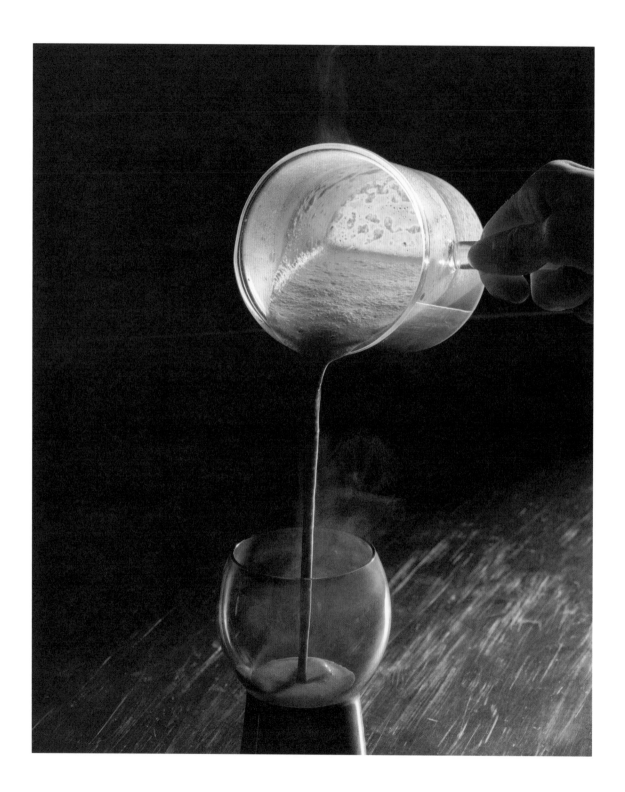

Sex Hot Chocolate

For stoking fires and desires...

Makes 1 tonic

1½ tablespoons cacao

1 pinch each of coriander, cardamom, and cayenne

⅛ teaspoon ground cinnamon

1 tablespoon Sex Butter (page 181)

1 cup milk, hot—I like Almond Milk (page 107)

3 drops stevia or 1 tablespoon raw honey

1

Combine all of the ingredients in the bowl of a blender and blend on high for 20 seconds.

2

Pour into a mug and sip sexy!

Horny Goat Weed Brownies

These fudgy, deeply chocolaty grain-free brownies get an extra hit from epimedium. I know it's time to make a batch when my chocolate drawer reaches max capacity (yes, I have one, and you can, too)—I go for dark chocolate that's 85% to 100%. Prepare the dry mix in advance, and you can have a fresh, warm batch in minutes. Another decadent option is to forgo the baking and form the dough into tablespoon-size truffles and roll them in cacao powder, cacao nibs, or chopped nuts or seeds. Store in the fridge for whenever you want a stimulating hit. Mucuna, ashwagandha, shatavari, cordyceps, eleuthero, and astragalus are all great options for these.

Makes 15 brownies

½ cup coconut oil or ghee

1 cup chopped dark chocolate (I prefer 85% to 100%)

3 tablespoons ground flaxseeds or 3 large eggs

2 cups almond butter

¼ cup maple syrup

1 tablespoon coconut butter

¾ cup cacao powder

1 teaspoon baking soda

Pinch of pink salt

3 teaspoons epimedium

1

Preheat the oven to 350°F. Line a 9 × 13-inch glass baking dish or cast-iron pan with parchment paper and set aside.

2

In a double boiler or a heatproof bowl set inside a simmering pot of water, combine the coconut oil and chocolate. Allow them to melt completely. Stir and set aside.

3

In a small bowl, if not using eggs, combine the flaxseeds with ½ cup plus 1 tablespoon water to make a paste.

4

In a large bowl, combine the melted chocolate, flaxseed paste or eggs, almond butter, maple syrup, and coconut butter. Stir until well incorporated.

5

In a medium bowl, sift together the cacao, baking soda, and salt. Stir in the epimedium. Whisk the dry ingredients into the wet ingredients until the batter is completely smooth. Pour the batter into the prepared baking dish and bake for 35 to 40 minutes, until a knife inserted in the center comes out gooey but not completely wet. Let the brownies cool completely before slicing. Store in a tightly sealed container at room temperature for up to 4 days.

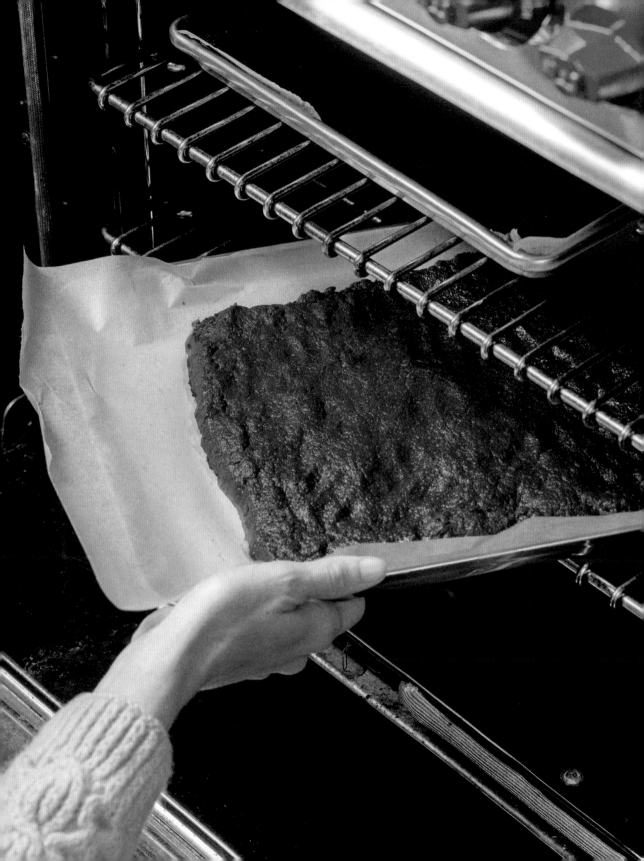

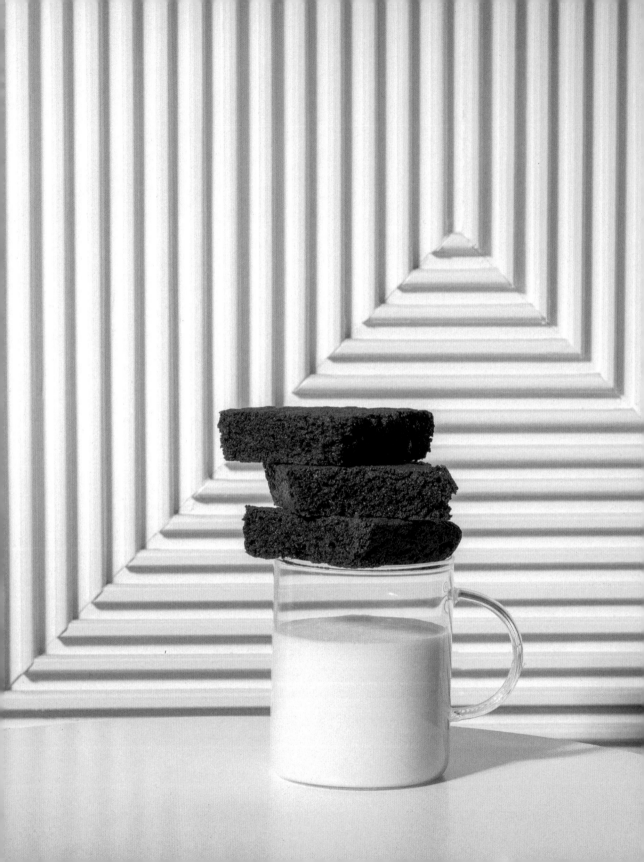

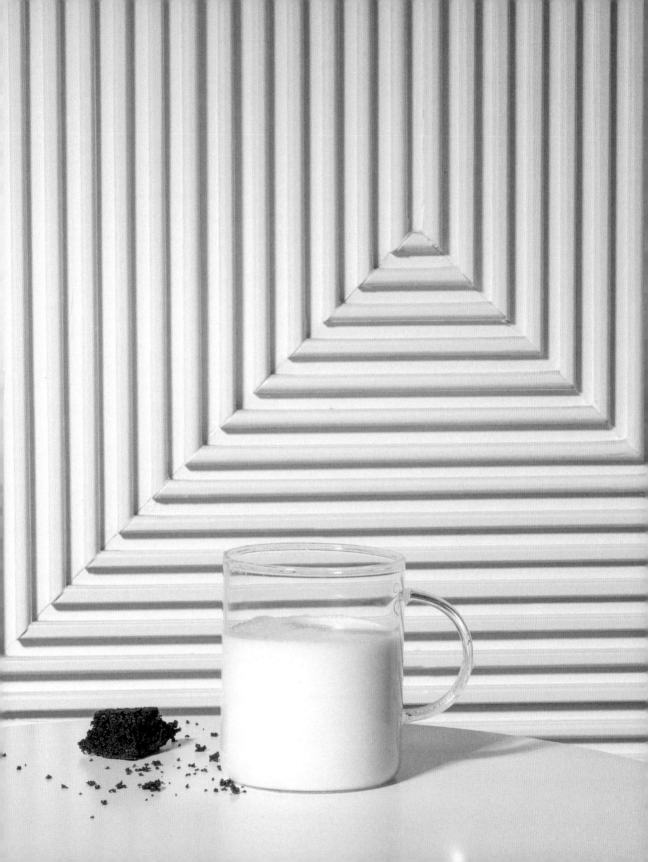

Shilajit Sex Drizzle

Magic shell for your fire! This rich chocolate sauce is intoxicating over ice cream, pancakes, fruit, or people. And definitely don't think twice about layering it over Horny Goat Weed Brownies (page 184) and a scoop of Shatavari Fig Ice Cream (page 191). If you really want to bump it up, invite all the sex adaptogens (epimedium, shatavari, and shilajit) to the affair. Other adaptogens to consider include ashwagandha, mucuna, reishi, cordyceps, eleuthero, ginseng, astragalus, and schisandra.

Makes about 2¼ cups

1½ cups cacao paste

¾ cup cacao butter

2 teaspoons coconut nectar

1 teaspoon shilajit

1 teaspoon raw vanilla bean powder or vanilla extract if you can't find raw powder

1

In a double boiler or a heatproof bowl set on top of a barely simmering pot of water, melt the cacao paste and cacao butter, stirring until uniform and silky.

2

Pour the melted mixture into the bowl of a blender, add the coconut nectar, shilajit, and vanilla, and blend until smooth.

3

Transfer to a shallow container to cool, then refrigerate until firm. Break into chunks and store at room temperature for up to 5 days or in the refrigerator in an airtight container for up to 6 months. Rewarm over a double boiler when ready to indulge.

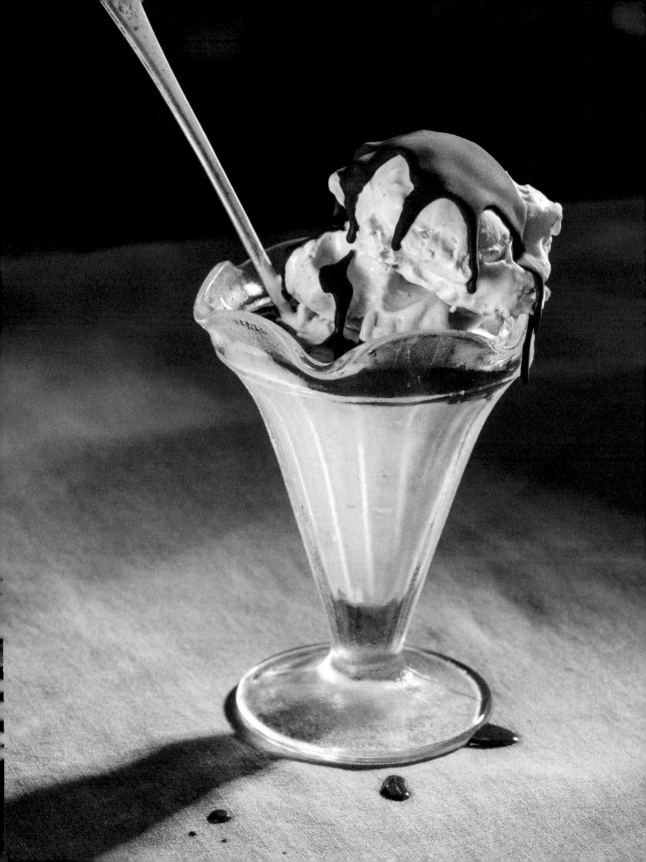

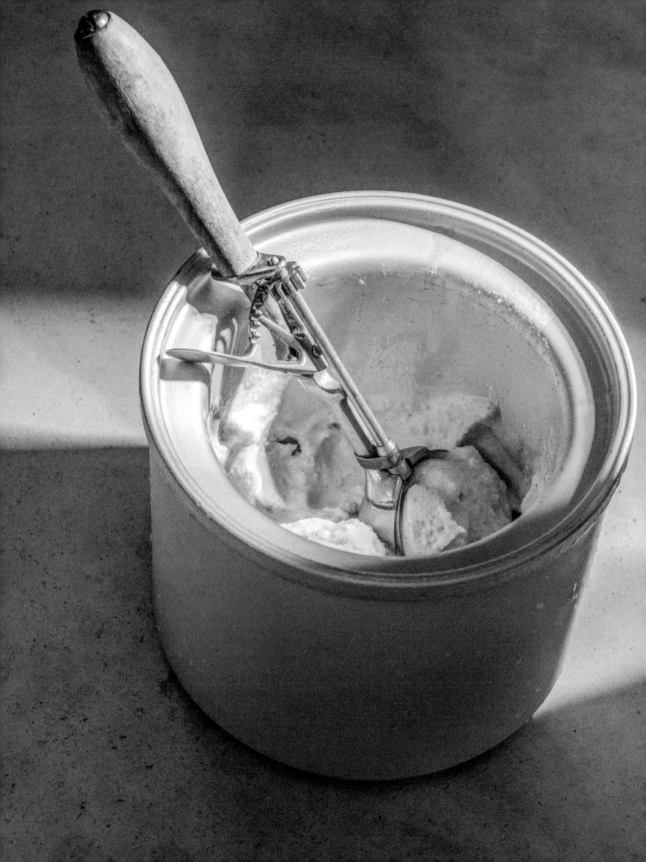

Shatavari Fig Ice Cream

I could eat this every day, straight out of the ice cream maker. I've also included variations for chocolate and strawberry, which means you can play with just about any adaptogens in the book. Mucuna, cordyceps, eleuthero, licorice, and shatavari play nicely with vanilla; reishi, ginseng, rhodiola, astragalus, eleuthero, and ashwagandha with chocolate; and schisandra with strawberry. Shilajit Sex Drizzle (page 188) accompaniment is strongly encouraged.

If you don't have an ice cream machine, make the base as called for here, pour into pop or ice cube molds, and freeze.

Serves 4

¾ cup dried Turkish figs

1½ cups coconut milk

2½ tablespoons shatavari

½ teaspoon raw vanilla bean powder or vanilla extract if you can't find raw powder

Pinch of pink salt

1

Fill a small bowl with ½ cup hot water. Add the figs and soak for 30 minutes, or for a few days in the refrigerator.

2

Combine the soaked figs, soaking water, coconut milk, shatavari, vanilla, and salt in a blender and pulse until just about smooth, leaving some of the fig seeds intact for pops of texture.

3

Pour the mixture into an ice cream maker and churn according to the manufacturer's instructions. Store in a mason jar or old ice cream container. Best enjoyed straight out of the blender or churner. For big batches, you may store them in the freezer for up to 1 month, but you will need to pull out and thaw them for 20 minutes to rescoop. Enjoy scooped over Horny Goat Weed Brownies (page 184) with a topping of Shilajit Sex Drizzle (page 188).

SPIRIT

BALANCE

Calm

Joy

Groundedness

Expansive Thoughts and Creativity

Contentedness

Stability

Patience and Tolerance

IMBALANCE

Depression

Anxiety

Lack of Patience

Obsession/Neurosis

Control Issues

Loss of Will

Irritability

Feeling Down or Blue

Racing Thoughts

Loss of Connection and/or Grounding

Overeating or Inability to Eat

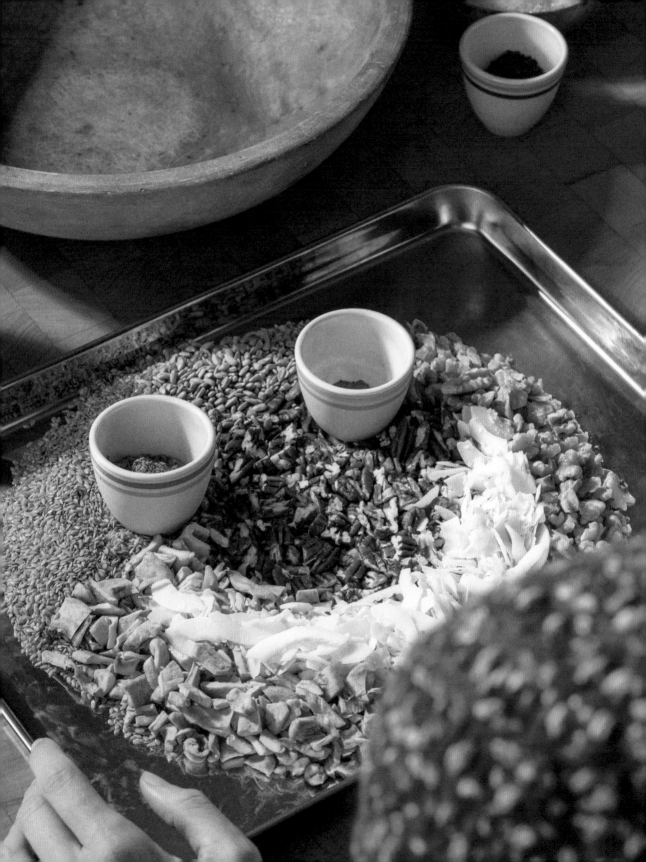

Our mood is directly connected to the quality of our inner life. When stress chemistry becomes chronic in the physical body, the emotional body is hit. That's when one might experience looping anxiety, cold depression, neurotic thinking, and overwhelming negativity. We can't pause life and its triggers, but we can upgrade the resilience of the mind and the spirit. One way to bolster ourselves is through herbs, especially reishi, whose name in TCM translates to "spiritual mushroom." It's described as a bridge between earth and heaven and is prized for its effects on consciousness; ashwagandha helps reduce tension and irritability and invites deeper mindfulness; and mucuna has been used for its bliss-boosting chemistry to open the heart for transformation.

The other powerful ally for a balanced resiliency is a spiritual practice. I've had a meditation practice for years, and it's made a difference in not only my day-to-day experience but connectedness to something bigger than myself, and faith in the whole process. I've found that when I don't use the practice, my capacity starts to wane. I feel overwhelmed by situations that seem outside of my control. When those thoughts come up, I can recognize that stress has built up in my system and has skewed my perspective. By managing stress with adaptogens and having time to tune in—to nature, or the energy within—I become the connectedness that re-centers my spirit.

I encourage you to find a practice that suits you. It could be a moment you carve out to be with your breath. It could be sitting with your eyes closed. It could be prayer in temple, your home, with a group, or with a partner. It doesn't need to be "meditation." You could call it a spiritual practice or a quiet time, or choose to never talk about it. It's not about doing it "right," it's about what works for you.

Ashwagandha

Ashwagandha is one of the most potent herbs for soothing symptoms of chronic stress. Traditionally it's used to sharpen minds, deepen clarity, and enhance meditative focus. Among Ayurveda practitioners, it remains a go-to for calming and lifting the spirits. Ashwagandha is a stamina-building anxiolytic, making it the perfect agent for tapping into the calm strength that already lives within you.

Min Daily Dose: ⅛ teaspoon (.13 gram)
Max Daily Dose: ½ teaspoon (.50 gram)
See also: Brain, Power

Reishi

Healers have long used this amazing mushroom for meditation. Reishi is perfect for attuning the mind, body, and spirit to higher function.

Min Daily Dose: 1 teaspoon (1.00 gram)
Max Daily Dose: 4 teaspoons (4.00 grams)
See also: Brain, Power

Mucuna

Mucuna's stimulation of dopamine production in the brain helps the mind and body relax. Mucuna is also a natural source of serotonin and tryptamine, both of which are soothing psychoactives that can aid the body in coping with anxiety and stress.

Min Daily Dose: 1/12 teaspoon (.23 gram)
Max Daily Dose: ½ teaspoon (1.00 gram)
See also: Brain, Sex

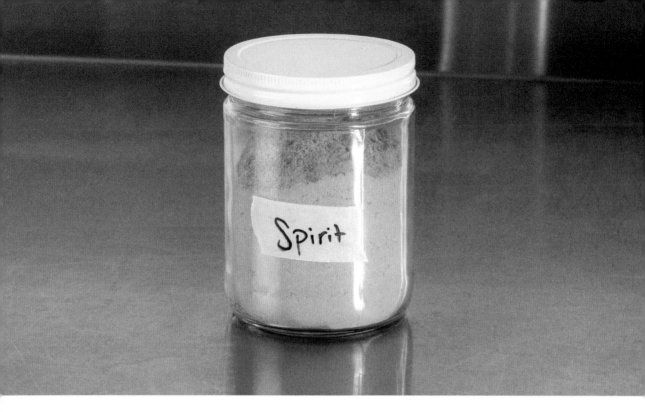

Spirit Mix

DAILY DOSE (1 serving)

⅛ teaspoon ashwagandha

½ teaspoon mucuna

1 teaspoon reishi

1
Combine the adaptogens in a small bowl and mix well.

BIG BATCH (30 servings)

3¾ teaspoons ashwagandha

5 tablespoons mucuna

½ cup plus 2 tablespoons reishi

1
Mix the adaptogens together and store in an airtight container for up to 1 year. Enjoy with water, tea, smoothies, or any other adaptogen-friendly recipe from this book.

2
Occasionally mix the batch to make sure the adaptogens are well combined.

Spirit Honey

You may eat this honey straight out of the jar or drizzled into granola, spread on toast, or as a honey ball rolled in cacao nibs. Use whenever you would like a little sweetness and an uplifting, adaptogenic hit.

DAILY DOSE (1 serving)

1¾ teaspoons Spirit Mix

2¼ teaspoons raw honey

1
Combine the adaptogens and honey in a small bowl and mix until a thick paste forms.

MONTH SUPPLY (30 servings)

1 Big Batch of Spirit Mix

1½ cups raw honey

1
Combine the adaptogens and honey in a medium bowl and mix with a rubber spatula until you have a thick, even paste. Transfer to a lidded glass jar and store at room temperature. Handled in a sanitary way (i.e., no double-dipping), this will last for up to 1 year.

Spirit Butter

Using this butter daily is a great assist for letting go of worry and finding ease with contentment. I use this in my hot tonic drinks and coffee, folded into baked goods, swirled into daal, or blended into a broth.

DAILY DOSE (1 serving)

1¾ teaspoons Spirit Mix

2¼ teaspoons ghee or coconut oil

1
Combine the adaptogens and ghee in a small bowl and mix until a smooth paste forms.

MONTH SUPPLY (30 servings)

1½ cups ghee or coconut oil

1 Big Batch of Spirit Mix

1
In a double boiler or a heatproof bowl set on top of a simmering pot of water, melt the ghee. Remove from the heat and stir in the adaptogens.

2
Let the mixture cool, then transfer to a lidded glass jar for storage. Stir occasionally as the mixture solidifies to ensure even distribution of the adaptogens. Store at room temperature for up to 1 year.

Holi Gold Chai

A soothing spirit salve with a dose of anti-inflammatory, mood-elevating turmeric.

Makes 1 tonic

1 cup milk, warmed—I like Almond Milk (page 107)

1 tablespoon Spirit Honey (page 197)

½ teaspoon ground turmeric

One 1-inch piece of ginger, peeled and coarsely chopped (about 1 tablespoon)

⅛ teaspoon raw vanilla bean powder

1/16 teaspoon ground cinnamon

Half of a whole clove or ⅛ teaspoon ground cloves

1 black peppercorn

Pinch of ground cardamom

1

Add all of the ingredients to the bowl of a blender and blend on high for 30 seconds. Sip in bliss!

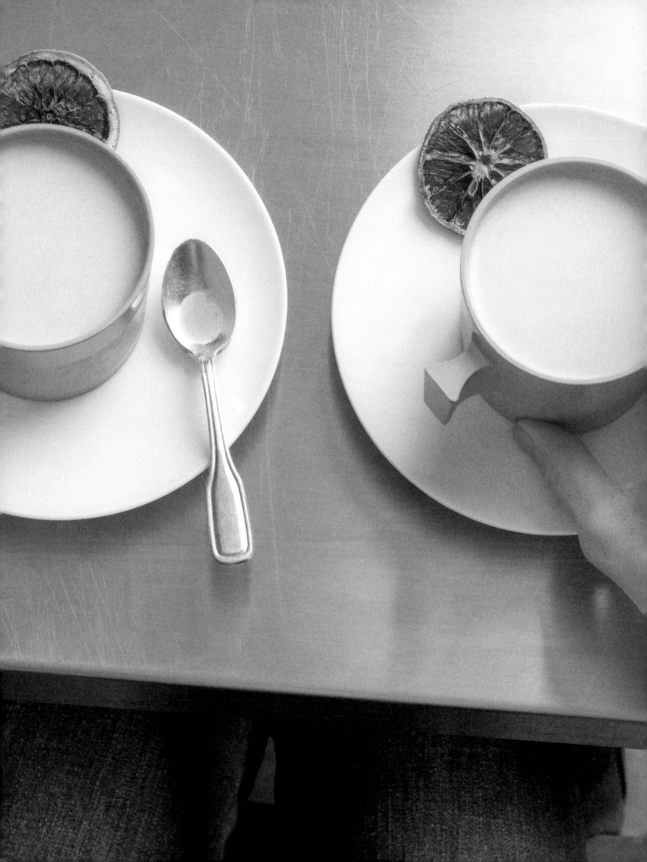

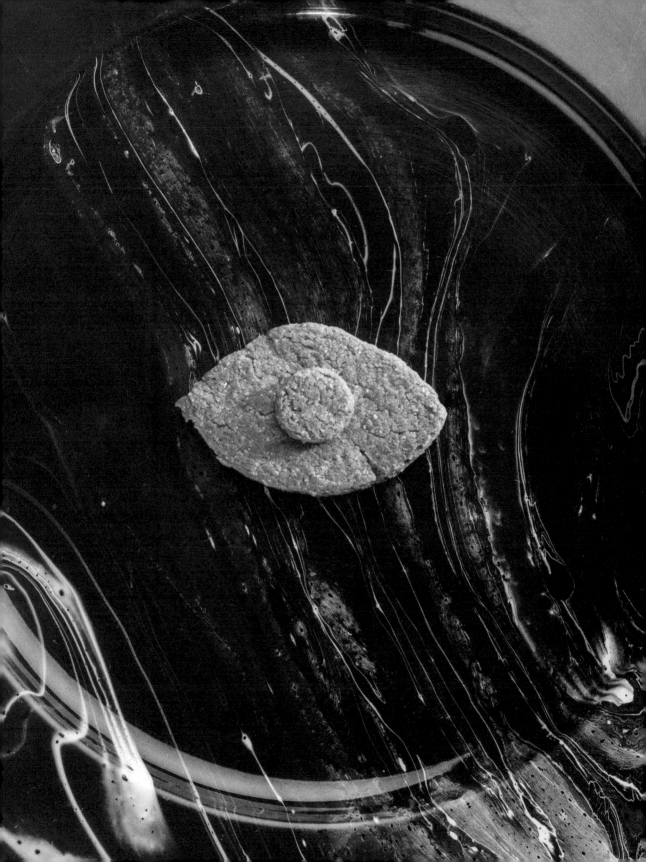

Spirit Snaps

A not too sweet, spiced, and elevating snack. I also love eating this dough raw and rolled into small balls dipped in chocolate.

Makes about 15 cookies

1½ cups almond flour

10 tablespoons arrowroot powder

1 teaspoon baking soda

Pinch of pink salt

1 teaspoon ground cinnamon

1 teaspoon raw vanilla bean powder or vanilla extract

10 tablespoons ashwagandha

½ teaspoon ground turmeric

10 tablespoons peeled and grated ginger

¼ cup coconut oil, melted

¼ cup maple syrup

1

Preheat the oven to 350°F. Line a baking sheet with parchment paper and set aside.

2

In the bowl of a food processor, mix the flour, arrowroot powder, baking soda, salt, cinnamon, vanilla, ashwagandha, and turmeric until well combined.

3

In a medium bowl, whisk together the ginger, coconut oil, and maple syrup. Add the wet ingredients to the food processor and pulse until the mixture forms a dough.

4

Form the dough into tablespoon-size balls and place them on the prepared baking sheet. For a crispier snap, gently press the dough to flatten, or leave thicker (more like a thumbprint) for a chewier consistency.

5

Bake for about 10 minutes, until the edges are golden. Let the cookies cool completely (ideally on a wire rack) before transferring them to a tightly sealed container. They can be stored, sealed, at room temperature for up to 1 week.

DR. PRATIMA RAICHUR

How do our thoughts impact our health?

Flexibility doesn't just pertain to the body. No matter what our individual circumstances in life may be, people with a healthy spirit will be flexible; they will be willing to accept, forgive, and let go when needed. Their mind will not be overly obsessive, they will be curious, they will laugh easily, and they will be peaceful and content.

From a holistic perspective, health and happiness come from a balance within the body, mind, and spirit. This balance is partially achieved through diet (including herbs) and exercise, but most importantly through attending to our thoughts. Thoughts create emotion, and emotions secrete hormones that affect both the mind and the body. Consistency of thoughts means that certain physiological patterns will persist, whether they are positive or negative. For this reason, it is critical that we include looking into our thought patterns and making sure they are beneficial, alongside any other wellness effort, like nutrition and exercise, in order to achieve genuine and lasting health and happiness.

Going deeper into health and happiness, Ayurveda believes that every soul has a purpose and that you won't fully be at peace until you know the purpose of your soul. We come to this earth with specific lessons to learn and fulfill and only when we live in accordance with our soul's purpose are we truly happy. So look deep within and ask yourself, What is my purpose and am I fulfilling it?

When you ask yourself this question, your mind may think of a certain hobby or passion. Is it possible to turn this into your work? Here's a little hint: If the rest of life blurs in the background when you're engaged with something, then you've discovered your soul's purpose.

DR. SARA GOTTFRIED

Does meditation affect brain function?

In my opinion, the brain is ultimately designed for mystic thought and action. When you look at the brains of nuns performing centering prayer, it's a highly evolved state of function. Meditators have bigger and more flexible brains than non-meditators. I love it when science supports the rich benefits of connecting to one's inner divinity.

Blissy Fig Balls

A dose of calming, magnesium-rich figs and mucuna perfect for your pocket, these sweet fruity drops are well suited for desks, lunch bags, and travel. You can either roll the dough into individual balls and store them in the fridge; or you could make a big batch of the dough, store it in the fridge for up to 1 month, and roll the balls out as desired (spiking with additional adaptogens if you're feeling it); or you could leave the adaptogens out of the dough recipe and add an adaptogen of the day or the week, per your wishes. This is one of the most versatile recipes in terms of being able to swap in other adaptogens. Try these with ashwagandha, reishi, shatavari, cordyceps, eleuthero, and astragalus.

Makes 16 balls

¾ cup dried Turkish figs

¼ cup dried mulberries or golden raisins

¼ cup pumpkin seeds

¼ cup sunflower seeds

1 teaspoon mucuna

Zest of 1 large orange, or 3 drops of orange essential oil

1 teaspoon raw vanilla bean powder

1

Combine the figs and mulberries in the bowl of a food processor and pulse until combined and a loose, granular dough forms. Add the pumpkin seeds, sunflower seeds, mucuna, orange zest, and vanilla and pulse until uniform.

2

Turn out the mixture on a parchment paper–lined work surface. Working with about 1 tablespoon at a time, squeeze the dough into balls—don't worry about them being too pretty; it's more about keeping them a uniform size for consistent dosage. There should be 16 balls altogether. Store them in a sealed container in the fridge for up to 2 weeks.

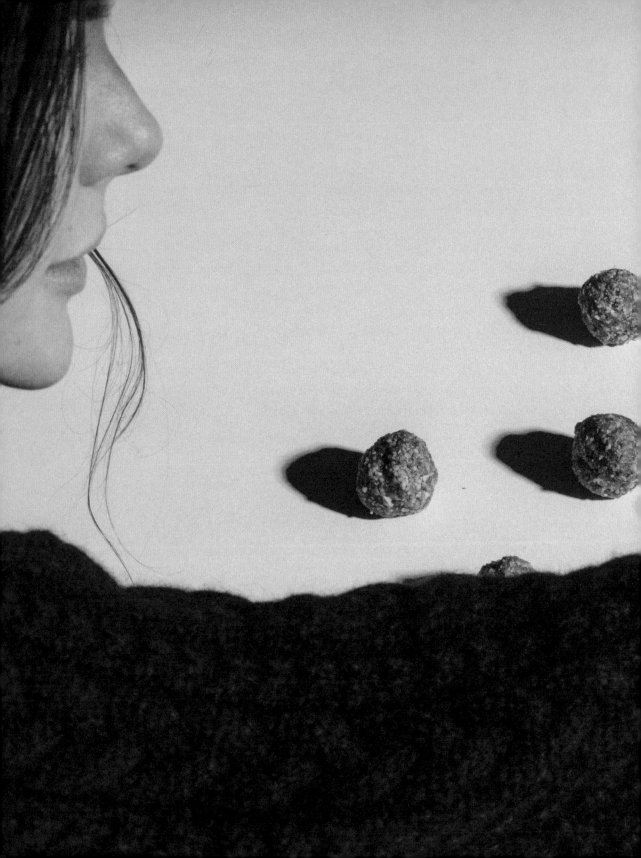

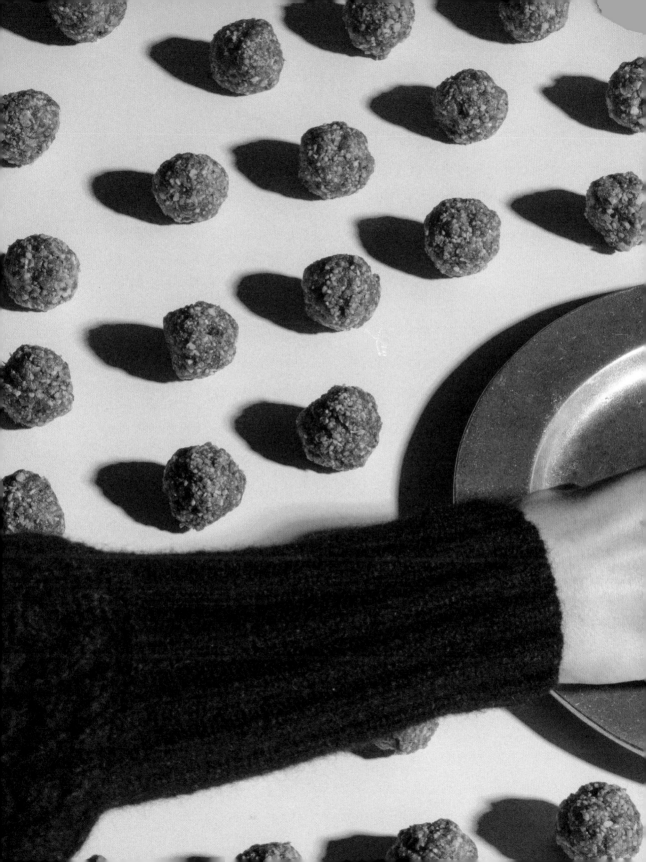

Spiced Apple Reishi Granola

This is another great recipe for big-batch preparation—just combine all of your nuts and seeds and store them in an airtight container for up to a year. Add adaptogens and wet ingredients when ready for takeoff. Other great adaptogens for mixing in include mucuna, ashwagandha, shatavari, cordyceps, eleuthero, and astragalus.

Serves 4

1⅓ cups dried apple rings (store-bought or homemade; gummy versions work better than crispy ones)

1 cup raw walnuts

1 cup raw pecans

½ cup flaxseeds

½ cup sunflower seeds

1 cup unsweetened and raw coconut flakes

¼ cup coconut oil, melted

¼ cup maple syrup

1 teaspoon reishi

10 teaspoons raw vanilla bean powder or vanilla extract if you can't find raw powder

1 teaspoon ground cinnamon

½ teaspoon pink salt

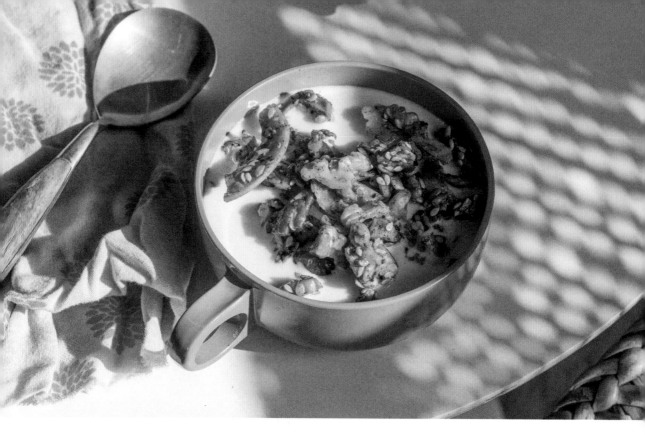

1

Preheat the oven to 350°F. Line a baking sheet or cast-iron pan with parchment paper and set aside.

2

Place the apple rings in the bowl of a food processor and pulse until the rings are in ¼-inch pieces. Transfer to a large mixing bowl.

3

Place the nuts in a food processor and pulse until broken into halves and quarters. Add to the mixing bowl.

4

Place the flaxseeds and sunflower seeds in the bowl of a food processor and pulse until broken into halves. Add them to the mixing bowl and sprinkle in the coconut flakes.

5

Drizzle the coconut oil and maple syrup over the mixture and stir to coat evenly. Add the reishi, vanilla, cinnamon, and salt and combine until evenly mixed.

6

Spread the granola over the baking sheet in an even layer and bake for 30 minutes, stirring every 10 minutes or so, until toasted and golden.

7

Allow the granola to cool completely before storing it an airtight container for up to 1 month.

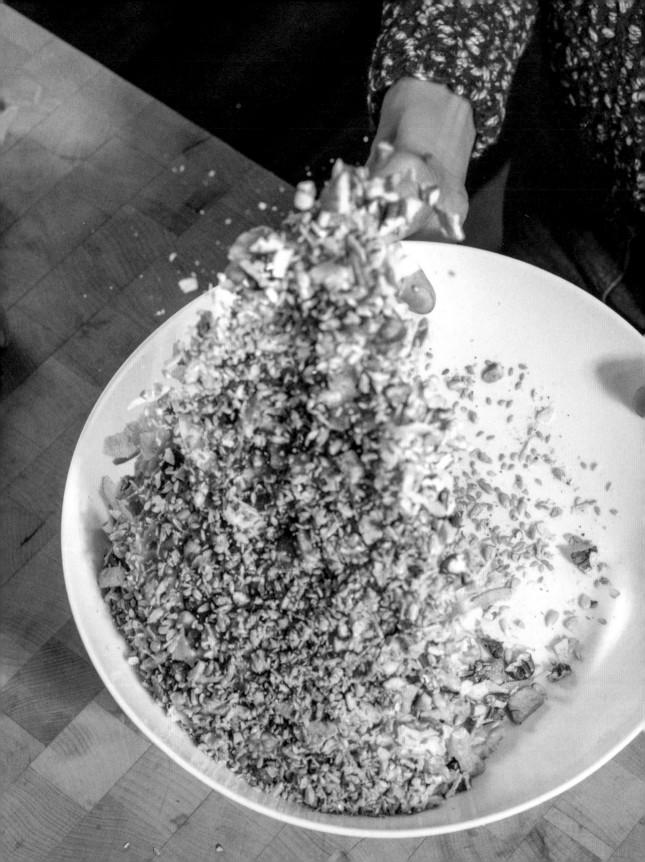

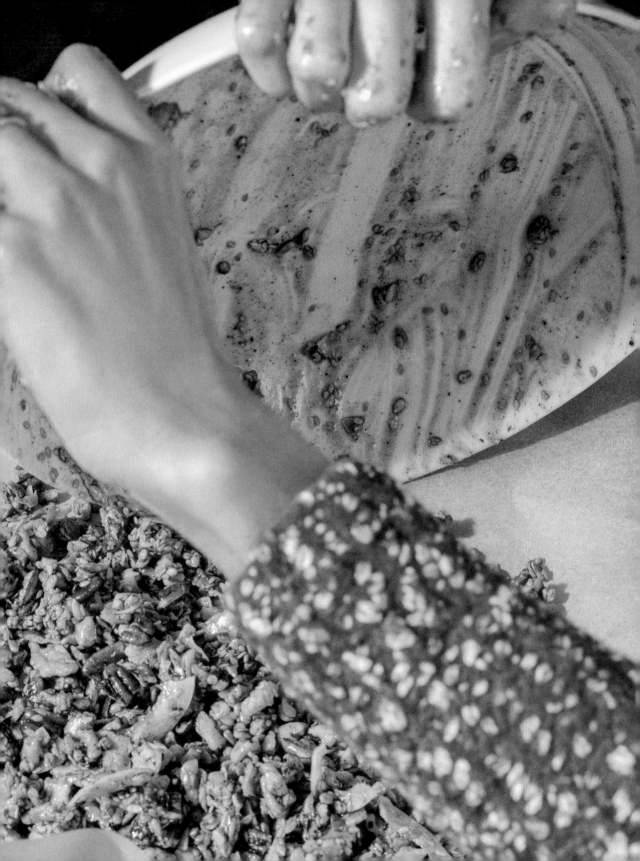

DREAM

BALANCE

Ability to Quiet Thoughts and Wind Down
Ability to Fall Asleep Quickly
Receiving Deep, Restful Sleep
Feeling Refreshed in the Morning

IMBALANCE

Feeling Tense or Wired
Inability to Fall Asleep or Stay Asleep

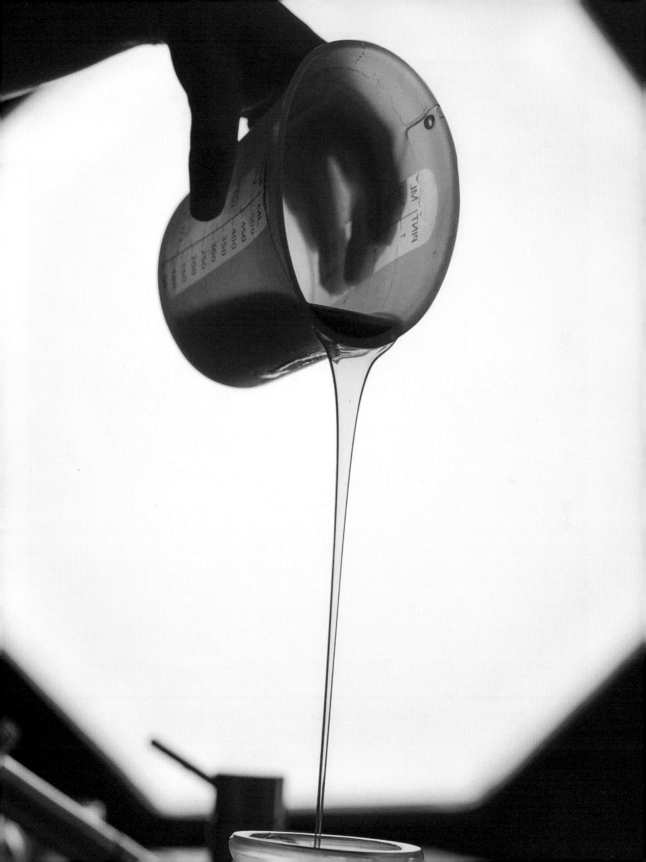

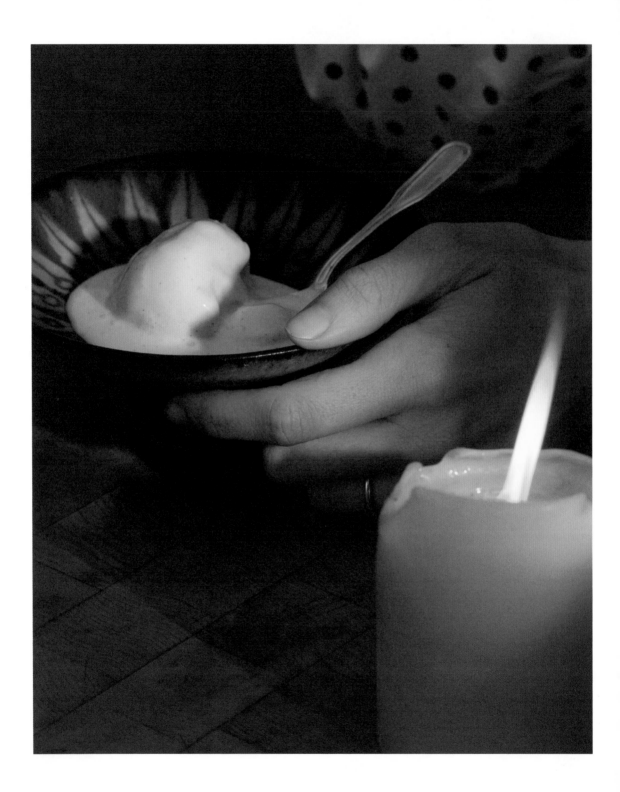

Sleep is at the heart of your mind, body, and spirit's health. You could take all the adaptogens in the world and partake in all the self-care practices and *still* not reach optimal resilience if you don't get the rest that you need—I know because I've been there. When my husband came into my life, he was horrified at how little sleep I was getting. He was right: I'd put it at the bottom of my priorities. Between staying up late to answer e-mails and then waking up early with a young child, I was getting four to six hours a night and had been for years, alongside a lot of travel.

I still managed to meditate twice a day, maintain a diet that was right for my body, surround myself with wonderful people, exercise, and have a job that I loved and felt connected to. I had life purpose…but I didn't have enough sleep. And all those other things only took me so far. It was really difficult for me to see that an underlying health issue could be solved by doing less and going to bed. I was investing all kinds of time and money in more extreme measures when all my body really wanted was decent, consistent sleep.

When my husband encouraged me to make sleep a priority, I was open to it. I immediately noticed that I could function so much better. All my physiological systems got to rest and reboot, and my subconscious got to experience its nocturnal unwind thanks to steady dream states. It was like rocket fuel that gave everything a boost—mood, clarity, patience, immunity, energy. It supported my parenting, my work, and my spiritual practice; and it radically changed my health, my stamina, and my decision-making. It also showed up in my blood work. It optimized my endocrine function and tamed inflammation I'd incurred as a result of my sleep deficit (coupled with exercise that was too aggressive for my system). In this way, sleep really is the master healer. Alongside herbs, functional foods, and a mindfulness practice, it is truly one of the pillars of success. The best part: It's *free* and it feels *good*.

Ashwagandha

In health, your cortisol levels will naturally decrease in preparation for sleep. But stress will overrule this rhythm, keeping cortisol levels elevated at night and disrupting sleep. Ashwagandha is incredible for regulating the production of cortisol while also revitalizing your life energy flow, which is the Ayurvedic key to being able to deeply rest.

Minimum daily dosage: ½ teaspoon (.13 gram)
Maximum daily dosage: 2 teaspoons (.50 gram)
See also: Brain, Power, Spirit

Licorice

As a tonic for both digestion and your adrenals, licorice is a potent sleep advocate, as raised cortisol and digestive deficiencies are interlinked with trouble settling down and staying asleep.

Minimum daily dosage: ⅛ teaspoon (.30 gram)
Maximum daily dosage: 1 teaspoon (1.6 grams)
See also: Power, Spirit

Reishi

Reishi is a promoter of healthy, deep sleep. It has been used in traditional Chinese medicine for its sedative action in those who suffer from restlessness, insomnia, palpitations, and other anxiety-related symptoms. Modern science now also confirms that reishi not only eases sleep but also increases sleep time.

Minimum daily dosage: 1 teaspoon (1.00 gram)
Maximum daily dosage: 4 teaspoons (4.00 grams)
See also: Brain, Power, Spirit

How Can We Get Better Sleep?

Start a ritual. One of the most effective things I started doing to get more sleep was to set a bedtime for myself. So at the very least, on the days when there's no time for any self-nourishment or attention, I can make sure that I'm getting into bed at a reasonable time. I'm not super rigid about it so it doesn't become something to be uptight about, but I find that it helps to set an alarm as a reminder when recalibrating your circadian rhythm. It's a cue to prepare a tonic, tea, or magnesium drink and turn off any electronics—and any other relaxing elements in my ritual to help bring a peaceful end of the day. You'll notice that over time your body will adapt to these habits and you won't need to set the alarms. Come evening tonic hour, my body knows it's that time. And when I turn in, it's because my body is happily inviting sleep and ready to drop the day.

Pass the Adaptogens

In Ayurveda, trouble sleeping is seen as a form of exhaustion itself, and the time-honored strategy to encourage sleep is not to sedate your already depleted body and mind, but rather balance and rejuvenate your system so it can achieve restorative sleep. Adaptogens are the ultimate sleep aid. Taken sometime after dinner—ideally about an hour before bed—sleep-suggesting adaptogens help your system wind down and your mind let go. Rather

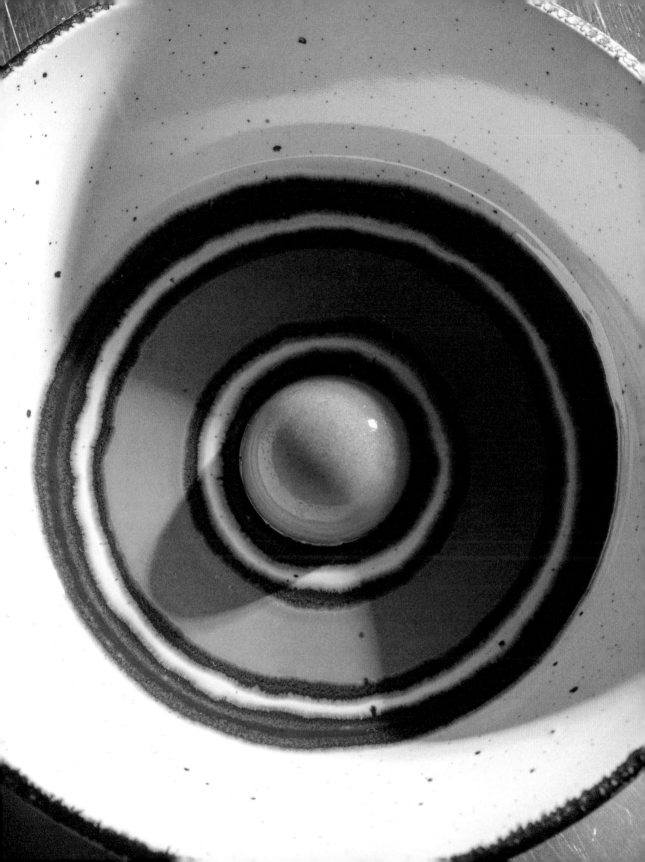

than act like sedatives, they recalibrate cortisol levels in the body, which is the main ingredient in helping you fall asleep more efficiently, stay asleep, and receive better quality sleep. In particular these three adaptogens—ashwagandha, licorice, and reishi—are incredible for regulating your sleep cycles and providing protection from disturbances. By calming the mind, settling the nervous system, and supporting what the body needs for deep rest and relaxation, they reduce the time it takes to fall asleep, help your body stay asleep, and improve sleep quality.

A Note on
Dream Recipes

Unlike "sleeping pills," these recipes will not knock you out and leave you groggy. You may enjoy these recipes at any time you feel like relaxing. They are best used regularly for a period of time to truly regulate your sleep.

DR. FRANK LIPMAN

Why is sleep crucial?

Sleep is something that most people are not getting enough of, yet it is essential for mental clarity and performance, a balanced mood, a strong immune system, a healthy stress response, proper cellular repair, and a vigorous metabolism. When you sleep, the body does much of its disease-fighting maintenance work.

DR. SARA GOTTFRIED

What are the benefits of regular deep sleep?

If you want to avoid a health breakdown, get fabulously restorative sleep. That's seven to eight and a half hours per night with the right balance of light, deep, and REM sleep. The biochemistry of chronic stress disrupts normal sleep by raising cortisol, making it hard to fall asleep or stay asleep, and harming blood sugar excursions, leading to early awakenings and weight-loss resistance. Sleep is when the lymphatic system shampoos your brain, removing toxins and debris, and when the wear-and-tear hormones (e.g., cortisol) are put back into balance with the growth-and-repair hormones (e.g., growth hormone). If you have too much cortisol and not enough growth hormone, you'll notice more skin wrinkling, facial aging, and chronic disease.

We need to get active about sleep. There's lots of talk about exercise, inner and outer beauty routines, and cultivating sexuality for reaching next-level wellness, but there are no such things as Brain, Sex, Spirit, and Beauty if there is no Dream. Conversely, when you invite sound, restful sleep into your life, all the nice things you do for yourself are amplified. You'll have a heightened ability to feel the effects of the adaptogens, you'll get buzzed from nourishing foods, and your meditation will take you to deeper depths than ever before. Sleep is also what helps us assimilate body and mind so that we can better receive connection and intimacy.

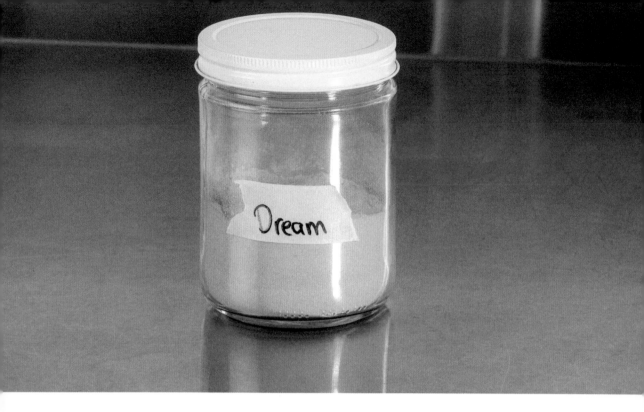

Dream Mix

DAILY DOSE (2 teaspoons)

½ teaspoon ashwagandha

1 teaspoon reishi

⅛ teaspoon licorice

1
Combine the adaptogens in a small bowl and mix well.

BIG BATCH (30 servings)

5 tablespoons ashwagandha

10 tablespoons reishi

3¾ teaspoons licorice

1
Mix the adaptogens together and store in an airtight container for up to 1 year. Enjoy with water, tea, smoothies, or any other adaptogen-friendly recipe from this book.

2
Occasionally mix the batch to make sure the adaptogens are well combined.

Dream Honey

Eat this honey straight out of the jar or use it wherever you'd like sweet adaptogenic calming. I like it in warmed milk, with tea, or drizzled over coconut butter for a tranquil treat.

DAILY DOSE

2 teaspoons Dream Mix

1 tablespoon raw honey

1
Combine the adaptogens and honey in a small bowl and mix until a thick paste forms.

MONTH SUPPLY

1 Big Batch of Dream Mix

1½ cups raw honey

1
Combine the adaptogens and honey in a medium bowl and mix with a rubber spatula until you have a thick, even paste.

2
Transfer to a lidded glass jar and store at room temperature. Handled in a sanitary way (i.e., no double-dipping), this will last for up to 1 year.

Dream Butter

DAILY DOSE

1¼ teaspoons Dream Mix

1 tablespoon coconut oil or ghee

1
Combine the adaptogens and coconut oil in a small bowl and mix until a smooth paste forms.

MONTH SUPPLY

½ cup coconut oil or ghee

1 Big Batch of Dream Mix

1
In a double boiler or a heatproof bowl set on top of a simmering pot of water, melt the coconut oil. Remove from the heat and stir in the adaptogens. Let the mixture cool, then transfer to a lidded glass jar for storage. Stir occasionally as the mixture solidifies to ensure even distribution of the adaptogens. Store at room temperature for up to 1 year.

Dream Tonic

This is a simple, yet life-changing evening ritual for you. Once you have made your big-batch dream honey (or feel free to use dream butter with a drop of stevia for a zero-sugar option), it's as simple as stirring or blending into warm milk. Don't be afraid to treat this as a "calm the F down" tonic and drink it during the day; it will not make you drowsy!

Makes 1 tonic

1 cup milk, gently warmed—I like Almond Milk (page 107)

1 tablespoon Dream Honey (page 219)

1

Combine the milk and adaptogens in the bowl of a blender and blend on high for 30 seconds.

2

Enjoy in a mug and begin to let the day go.

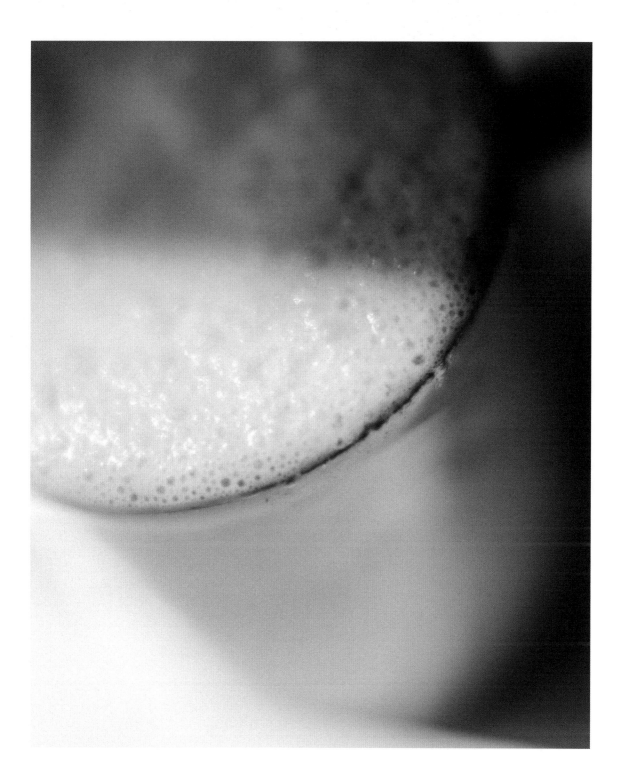

Dream 223

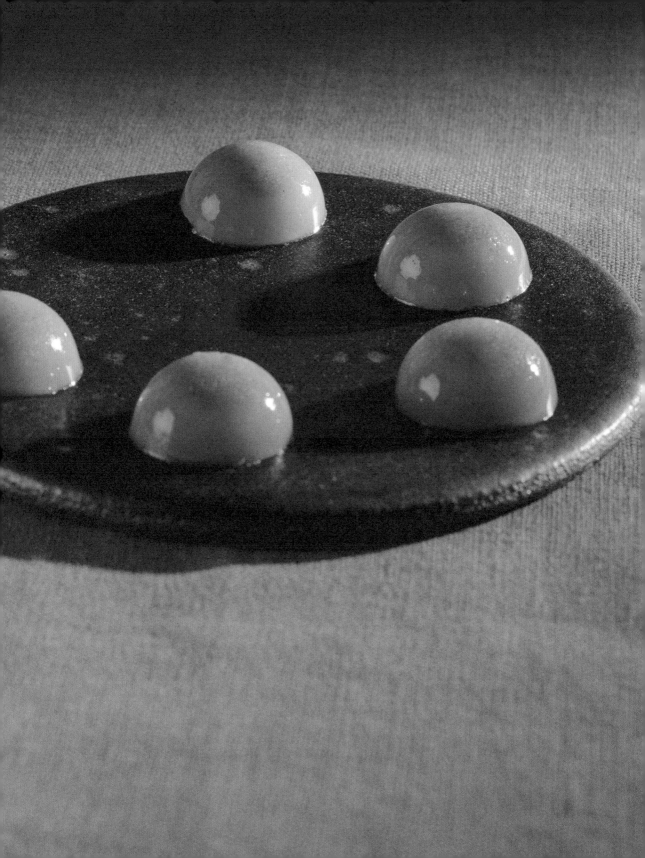

Ashwagandha Cider Jellies

These jellies are like a glass of mulled tea before bed with warming ginger, cardamom, and cinnamon. They could also be made with reishi, cordyceps, shatavari, mucuna, eleuthero, and astragalus. Feel free to use gelatin in place of agar-agar if it's your preference.

Makes twenty 2-ounce jellies

2 cups apple juice

1 teaspoon ground ginger

1 teaspoon ground turmeric

½ teaspoon ground cinnamon

¼ teaspoon ground cardamom

3 tablespoons agar-agar

3 teaspoons ashwagandha

1

In a small saucepan over medium-low heat, bring the apple juice to a simmer. Add the ginger, turmeric, cinnamon, and cardamom and stir. Cover the saucepan and let simmer for 10 minutes for the flavors to infuse.

2

Remove the saucepan from the heat and strain the mixture. Discard the residue and pour the liquid back into the saucepan. At this point, you could allow the cider to cool, stir in the ashwagandha, and have a batch of dusted apple cider to sip on. To continue with the jellies, bring the saucepan to a simmer over medium-low heat. Whisk in the agar-agar and continue to whisk for 5 minutes as the mixture simmers. The agar-agar should be completely dissolved and you'll now have closer to 1½ cups of liquid.

3

Place the mixture in the bowl of a blender. Add the ashwagandha and blend on low for 10 seconds. The higher and longer you blend, the more air in the mixture, leading to bubbly jellies. Tap the blender base on the counter a few times to release any trapped air. Pour the mixture into 2-ounce candy molds, ice cube trays, or a small baking dish lined with parchment paper and chill in the fridge for a minimum of 1 hour, until set. If using a lined baking dish, slice the jellies into ½-inch squares once they are set. Store in the fridge for up to 1 week.

Iced Licorice Cream

Sweet, rich, and malty, this coconut-based ice cream is cloudlike and fluffy. This recipe will certainly soothe your nighttime ritual, but it won't knock you out, so feel free to enjoy whenever the mood strikes—particularly those of you looking to nourish your adrenals. Consider adding Blue Roman chamomile essential oils to increase the calming factor. Other adaptogens that would work well here are schisandra, amla, eleuthero, astragalus, and shatavari.

If you don't have an ice cream machine, make the base as called for here, pour it into pop or ice cube molds, and freeze.

Makes 2½ cups

2 cups coconut cream
(from the can is all good)

2 teaspoons licorice

1 teaspoon raw vanilla bean powder or vanilla extract if you can't find raw powder

1

Combine all of the ingredients in the bowl of a blender and blend for 20 seconds. Pour the mixture into an ice cream maker. Churn for about 8 minutes, until ice cream consistency.

2

You can store the ice cream in a 9 × 5-inch loaf pan, a to-go coffee mug, or a clean empty ice cream carton. It's best enjoyed straight out of the blender or churner. For big batches, you may store it in the freezer for up to 1 month, but you will need to pull it out and thaw it for 20 minutes to rescoop.

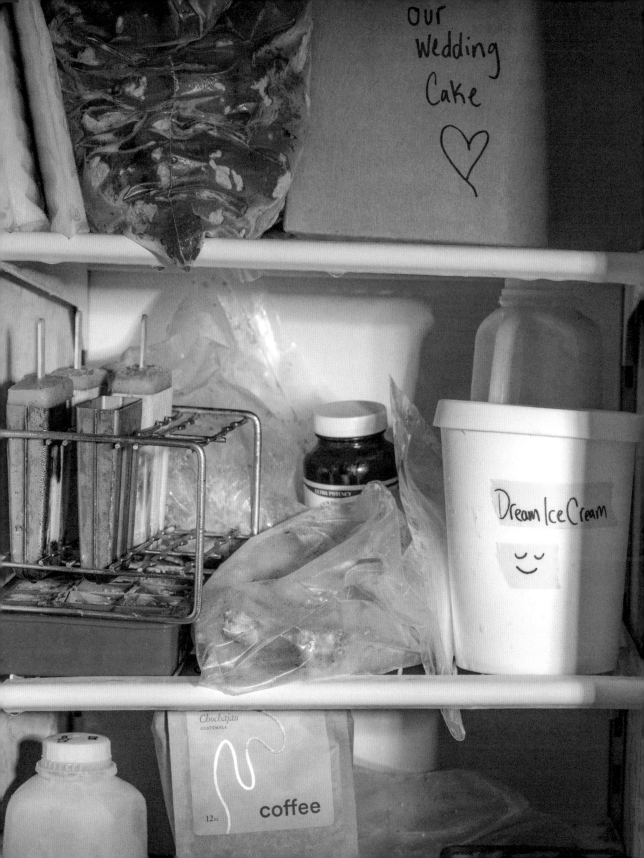

Reishi Banana Bread

This sticky bun–like loaf is mineralizing, relaxing, and the perfect comfort food. Sliced, warmed, and anointed with Dream Butter (page 219) or Dream Honey (page 219), it is a good night to all. It would also pair perfectly with your Dream Tonic (page 220) or, because reishi is a noteworthy Brain adaptogen, you could hook it up with your Brainy Coffee (page 138) in the morning or enjoy it as an afternoon brain snack. Make a batch for the week and reheat it before each meal! Try this recipe with mucuna, shatavari, cordyceps, eleuthero, and astragalus.

Serves 6

1 tablespoon ground flaxseeds

2 cups overripe bananas

½ cup coconut oil, melted

¼ cup maple syrup

1½ cups almond flour

½ cup tapioca flour

1 teaspoon vanilla bean powder

½ teaspoon baking soda

½ teaspoon pink salt

2 tablespoons reishi

1

Preheat the oven to 350°F.

2

In a large bowl, mix the flaxseeds with 3 tablespoons water to make a smooth, viscous slurry. Stir in the bananas, coconut oil, and maple syrup.

3

In another large bowl, mix together the almond flour, tapioca flour, vanilla bean powder, baking soda, salt, and reishi until just combined. Add the dry ingredients to the wet ingredients and mix until the batter is smooth.

4

Pour the batter into small cake molds or loaf pans and bake for 35 minutes, or until a knife inserted in the center comes out clean. Eat piping hot or store the bread at room temperature or in the fridge in a lidded container or zip-top bag for up to 5 days.

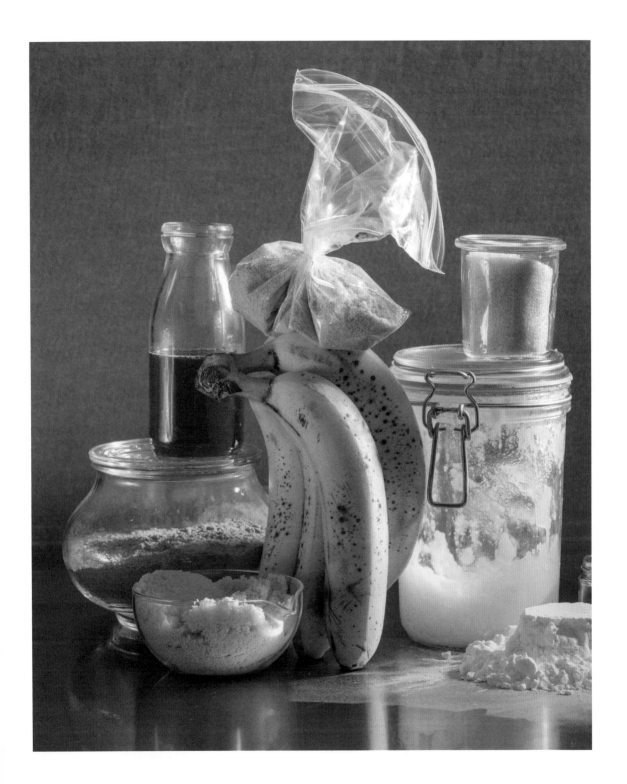

Dream

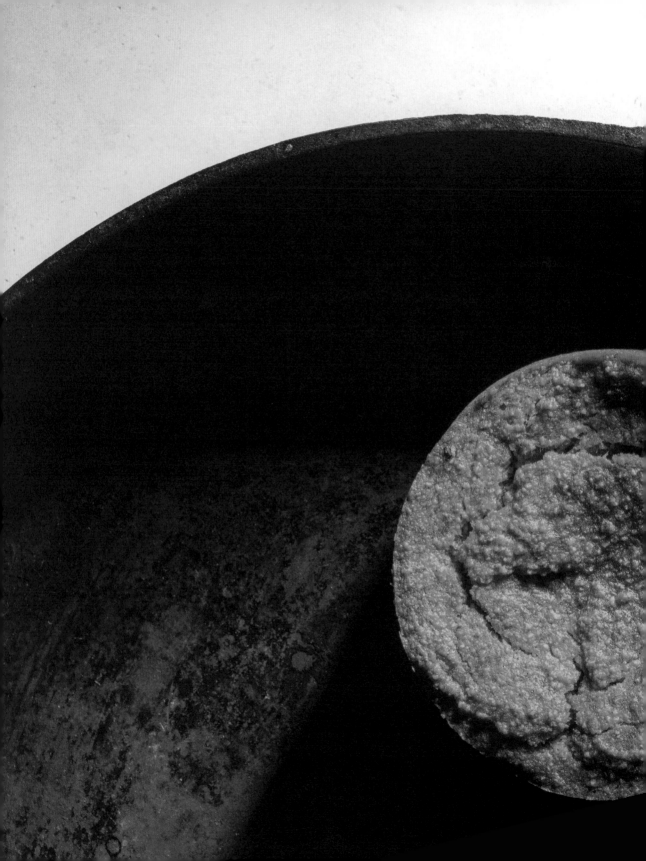

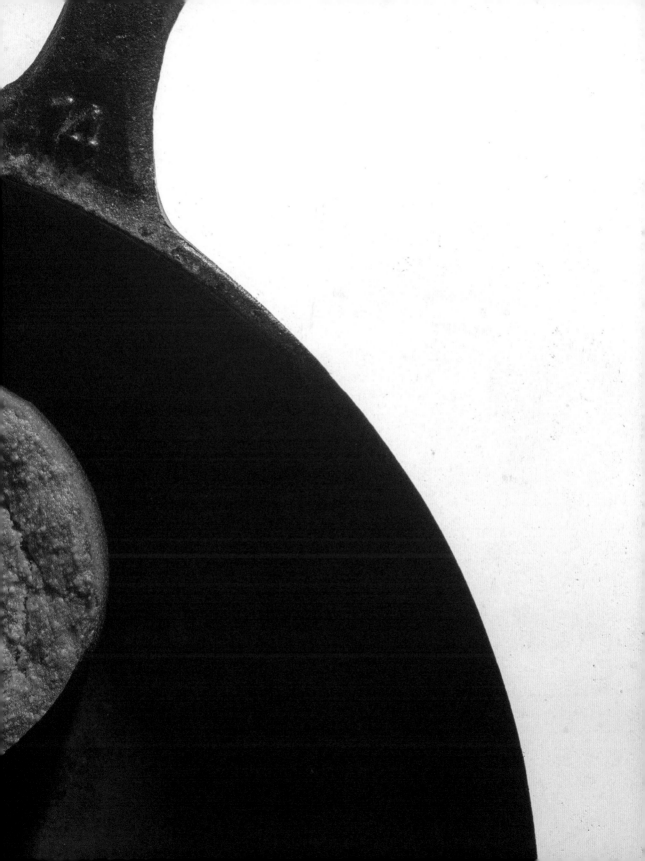

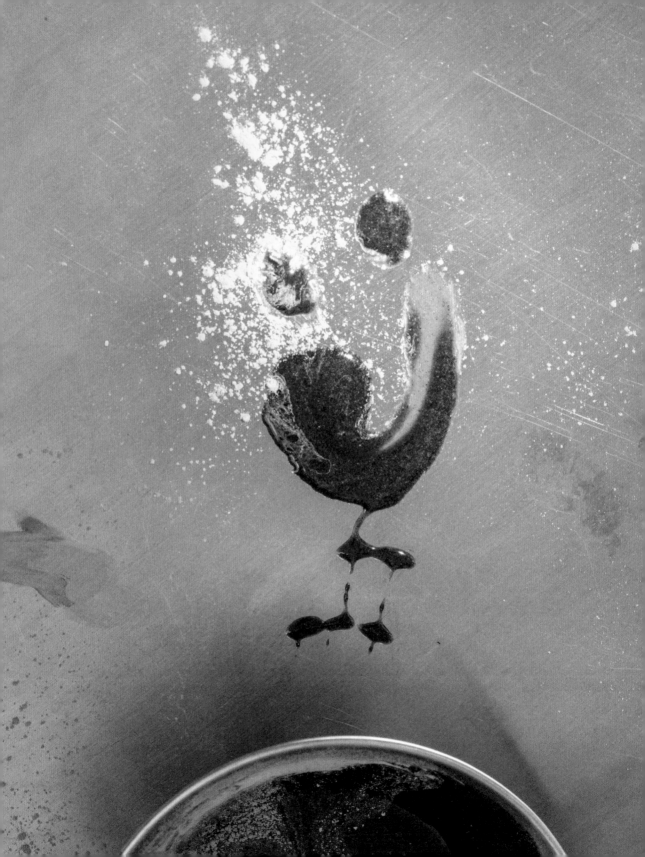

ENDNOTES

1
Astragalus houses three types of active compounds: http://www.mdpi.com/1420 -3049/19/11/18850/htm.

2
Saponins are thought to lower cholesterol: https://www.ncbi .nlm.nih.gov/pmc/articles /PMC2928447/.

3
which can help prevent heart disease, cancer, and immunodeficiency viruses: https://www.ncbi.nlm.nih.gov /pubmed/15678717.

4
considered to have antimicrobial, antiviral, and anti-inflammatory properties: https://www.ncbi.nlm.nih.gov /pubmed/22909979.

5
particularly beneficial for supporting the immune system: https://www.ncbi.nlm.nih.gov /pubmed/22981502.

6
called upon to quell infections and viruses: http://www. huffingtonpost.ca/2014/12 /08/what-is-Astragalus_n_ 6289286.html.

7
beat back disease-causing inflammation: https://www.ncbi .nlm.nih.gov/pubmed /26916911.

8
protect the cardiovascular system: https://www.ncbi.nlm.nih .gov/pubmed/25098261.

9
regulate or prevent diabetes: https://www.ncbi.nlm.nih.gov /pmc/articles/PMC3855992/.

10
support the renal system: https://www.ncbi.nlm.nih.gov /pubmed/19735713.

11
boosting your immune system: https://www.ncbi.nlm.nih.gov /pmc/articles/PMC3110835/.

12
helping athletes take on tougher and longer feats: https://www .ncbi.nlm.nih.gov/books /NBK92758/

13
similar effects to prescription drugs like Viagra: https://www .ncbi.nlm.nih.gov/pubmed /17499557.

ACKNOWLEDGMENTS

Rachel Holtzman, thank you for your organization and talent. It was no small feat untangling the ball of yarn in my head.

Heather Scott, thank you for understanding the way that everything needs to be.

Nastassia Brückner, a thank-you for your natural eye and organic storytelling.

Nicole Tourtelot, thank you for championing this work and getting it out there; it's been a long and winding road.

Lucia Watson, thank you for having faith in the vision and supporting us every step of the way.

Amy Wilson and Lauren Schaefer, thank you for your talents and presence.

INDEX

Note: Page numbers in **bold** refer to primary treatments of the adaptogen.

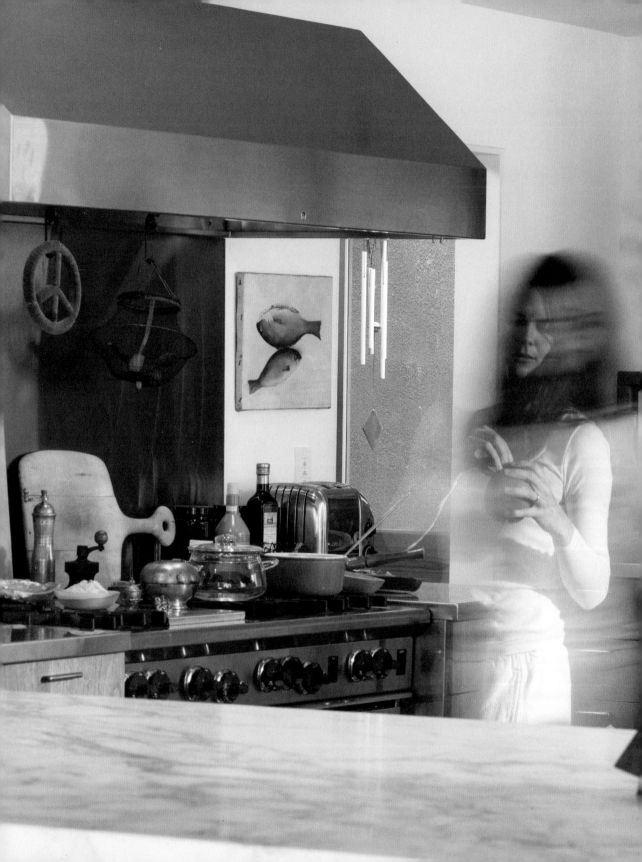